D1238776

BOTTOM LINE'S GUIDE TO
HEALTHY AGING

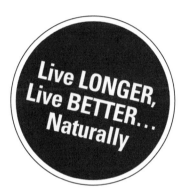

Live LONGER,
Live BETTER...
Naturally

B

BottomLineBooks

BottomLineInc.com

Contents

5. AGE WELL IN YOUR HOME

6. SECRETS TO STAYING STEADY ON YOUR FEET

7. DRIVE SAFER LONGER

8. MEDICATION SMARTS

9. HEALTHFUL EYES, EARS, NOSE AND MOUTH

10. HELP FOR CHRONIC CONDITIONS

11. BRAIN AND MEMORY HEALTH

12. HEART HEALTH AND STROKE

13. LIVE CANCER FREE

14. MIND AND BODY

CHAPTER 1

Live Longer and Better

Anti-Aging Secrets from the Renowned Canyon Ranch

Mark Liponis, MD, corporate medical director of the Canyon Ranch Health Resorts in Tucson, Arizona, and Lenox, Massachusetts. He is the author of *Ultralongevity* and coauthor of *Ultraprevention*.

Scientists still haven't figured out exactly what causes aging. Is it due to oxidation (a natural process that damages the body's cells)? Genetics? Wear and tear from daily living and environmental assaults? Or perhaps the gradual weakening of the immune system?

Recent thinking: An overactive immune system can contribute to premature aging.

Sound far-fetched? This belief stems, in part, from exciting research on biological factors that influence disease and the aging process. *Consider these facts...*

Immunity and Aging

A healthy adult's immune system is composed of 30 billion to 50 billion white blood cells that are equipped with powerful molecular weapons to destroy disease-causing bacteria, viruses and fungi. But if that army of white blood cells becomes overactive due to exposure to an excess of those germs, it can cause "collateral" damage that produces aging.

According to this theory, overactive white blood cells chew up neurons in the brain (Alzheimer's disease)...eat through the lining of arteries (heart disease)...and attack cartilage in the joints (arthritis).

An overactive immune system also produces an overabundance of antibodies (proteins in the body that help fight infection). Instead of fighting microbial enemies, these antibodies attack one or more of the body's organs.

A Healthy Immune System

Dozens of studies have shown that the following steps can help prevent the immune system from becoming overactive…

1. Breathe deeply. Diseases that interfere with normal breathing, such as asthma, bronchitis and sleep apnea (temporary cessation of breathing during sleep), cause an increase in immune activity.

But breathing also is impeded even in people without respiratory disease. It's common to breathe shallowly whenever you're preoccupied—while driving the car, for example, or balancing your checkbook.

Simple step: Become aware of and deepen your breathing.

What to do: Fold your arms across your belly while you're sitting. With each breath in, your arms should rise. That means your abdomen is expanding and you're performing "abdominal breathing"—relaxed, deep breathing that calms your immune system. If your arms don't move up, or they move inward, you need to focus on relaxing and expanding your belly with each breath.

Practice this breathing technique for 15 minutes, once a day. Eventually, you will become more mindful of your breathing during everyday activities.

2. Eat small meals. Eating is stressful for the immune system because it has to filter every substance swallowed to check for potentially harmful bacteria, viruses and other germs, then gear up to defend against them. The bigger the meal, the greater the stress.

Simple step: Instead of eating three large meals, eat small meals every few hours—breakfast, a mid-morning snack, lunch, a midday snack and dinner. Have a half cup of soup, not a whole cup. Eat half a sandwich. Snack on a handful of nuts. For small meals, high-fiber foods (such as whole grains, beans, fruits, vegetables, nuts and seeds) work best—they're quickly filling and digest slowly, which delays hunger.

3. Get high-quality sleep. Studies of people who have voluntarily stayed awake for up to 80 hours have shown that sleep deprivation can increase CRP levels fivefold. But sleep quality—deep, restful sleep—is as important as the amount of time you spend in bed.

How do you know that you're getting quality sleep? *Ask yourself these questions…*

- Do I often fall asleep when I'm reading or watching TV?
- Do I have to catch up on sleep during weekends?
- Do I wake up most mornings feeling tired?

If you answered "yes" to any of these questions, you may not be getting enough quality sleep.

Simple step: Try a "sleep mantra"—an image, thought or feeling on which to focus—to help clear your mind of disturbing thoughts so that you can peacefully drift off into deep, restful sleep.

Examples: Repeat a phrase, such as "I am so happy to be in bed"…focus on a happy memory from the past…or think about someone you love. Even if you suffer from serious insomnia, this technique can be part of your treatment plan.

4. Try dancing (or other "rhythmic" activities). People who exercise rhythmically—such as by dancing, swimming, rowing or walking to music—have lower levels of immune activation than people who do not exercise this way, such as golfers or tennis players. No one knows why, but perhaps rhythmic exercise synchronizes with the natural rhythms of the body, such as the heartbeat and breathing.

Simple step: For beginners (people who have not been active), try walking at a steady pace while listening to music…swimming…ballroom dancing… or basic aerobics. Intermediates may want to try biking…rowing…jumping rope…or tap, hip-hop or square dancing. For those who are advanced, good choices include rhythmic martial arts (such as karate, tae kwon do, jujitsu and tai chi)…hiking…or strenuous dance forms, such as jitterbug, African dance or polka.

5. Forge strong emotional connections. When you experience deep emotional bonds, such as love for your spouse, children, friends or pets, you are less likely to feel the negative emotions of anxiety, hostility or depression—all of which researchers have linked to an overactive immune system.

Simple step: Keep a daily diary of incidents that reflect your emotional connections.

Examples: Write about an enjoyable phone conversation with a friend… special time spent with your children…or playing Frisbee with your dog in the park. Whenever you feel anxious, angry or sad, open the journal, read it—and remind yourself about the love in your life.

6. Create a soothing environment. Anecdotal evidence suggests that the immune system doesn't like a noisy, chaotic or stressful environment. It prefers an "outside world" that's nurturing and calm.

Simple steps: Play music that relaxes you. Display artwork that you enjoy looking at. Bring wonderful smells, such as fresh flowers or mulled apple cider, into your home.

7. Get your nutrients. Nutritional supplements can help calm an overactive immune system. See a nutritionist for advice on the supplements that are right for you.

Simple step: Take your multivitamin about an hour before your biggest meal of the day. This helps reduce the immune activity that is triggered after you eat.

You Can Have a Much Younger Body and Mind—A Few Simple Changes Can Turn Back the Clock

Mike Moreno, MD, who practices family medicine in San Diego, where he is on the board of the San Diego Chapter of the American Academy of Family Physicians. He is also the author of *The 17 Day Plan to Stop Aging.* DrMikeDiet.com

What is it that allows some people to remain robust and healthy well into their 80s and 90s while others become frail or virtually incapacitated? It's not just luck. New studies indicate that aging is largely determined by controllable factors.

Case in point: Millions of people have chronic inflammation, which has been linked to practically every "age-related" disease, including arthritis, heart disease and dementia.

Inflammation can usually be controlled with stress management, a healthful diet, weight loss (if needed) and other lifestyle changes, but there are other, even simpler, steps that can strengthen your body and brain so that they perform at the levels of a much younger person.

To turn back your biological clock…

Challenge Your Lungs

You shouldn't be short of breath when you climb a flight of stairs or have sex, but many adults find that they have more trouble breathing as they age—even if they don't have asthma or other lung diseases.

Why: The lungs tend to lose elasticity over time, particularly if you smoke or live in an area with high air pollution. "Stiff" lungs cannot move air efficiently and cause breathing difficulty.

Simple thing you can do: Breathe slowly in and out through a drinking straw for two to three minutes, once or twice daily. Breathe only through your mouth, not your nose. This stretches the lungs, increases lung capacity and improves lung function.

Helpful: Start with an extra-wide straw, and go to a regular straw as you get used to breathing this way.

Drink Thyme Tea

When the lungs do not expand and contract normally (see above), or when the tissues are unusually dry, you're more likely to get colds or other infections, including pneumonia. The herb thyme contains thymol, an antioxidant that may help prevent colds, bronchitis and pneumonia and soothe chronic respiratory problems such as asthma, allergies and emphysema.

Simple thing you can do: Add a cup of thyme tea to your daily routine. If you have a chronic or acute respiratory illness, drink two cups of thyme tea daily—one in the morning and one at night.

To make thyme tea: Steep one tablespoon of dried thyme (or two tablespoons of fresh thyme) in two cups of hot water for five minutes, or use thyme tea bags (available at most health-food stores).

If you take a blood thinner: Talk to your doctor before using thyme—it can increase risk for bleeding. Also, if you're allergic to oregano, you're probably allergic to thyme.

Another simple step: Drink at least six to eight eight-ounce glasses of water every day. This helps loosen lung mucus and flushes out irritants, such as bacteria and viruses.

Lower Your Heart Rate

Heart disease is the leading cause of death in the US. The average American would live at least a decade longer if his/her heart pumped blood more efficiently.

Elite athletes typically have a resting heart rate of about 40 beats a minute, which is about half as fast as the average adult's resting heart rate. This reduced heart rate translates into lower blood pressure, healthier arteries and a much lower rate of heart disease. But you don't have to be an athlete to lower your heart rate—you just have to get a reasonable amount of aerobic exercise.

Simple thing you can do: Aim for a resting heart rate of 50 to 70 beats a minute—a good range for most adults. To do this, get 30 minutes of aerobic exercise, five days a week. Good aerobic workouts include fast walking, bicycling and swimming. Even if you're not in great shape, regular workouts will lower your resting heart rate.

To check your pulse: Put your index and middle fingers on the carotid artery in your neck, and count the beats for 15 seconds, then multiply by four. Check your pulse before, during and after exercise.

Walk Just a Little Faster

A study published in *The Journal of the American Medical Association* found that people who walked faster (at least 2.25 miles per hour) lived longer than those who walked more slowly.

Why: Faster walking not only lowers your heart rate and blood pressure but also improves cholesterol and inhibits blood clots, the cause of most heart attacks.

Simple thing you can do: You don't have to be a speed-walker, but every time you go for a walk, or even when you're walking during the normal course of your day, increase your speed and distance slightly.

Time yourself and measure your distance to monitor your progress, and create new goals every two weeks. Walk as fast as you can but at a speed that still allows you to talk without gasping, or if you're alone, you should be able to whistle. You'll notice improvements in stamina and overall energy within about two to three weeks.

Shake Up Your Mental Routines

In a study of about 3,000 older adults, those who performed mentally challenging tasks, such as memorizing a shopping list or surfing the Internet to research a complex topic, were found to have cognitive skills that were the typical equivalent of someone 10 years younger. You'll get the same benefit from other activities that promote thinking and concentration.

Why: These tasks trigger the development of new neurons in the brain, which boost cognitive function.

Simple thing you can do: Try to change your mental routines daily.

Fun ideas: If you're right-handed, use your left hand to write a note. Study the license number of the car in front of you, and see if you can remember it five minutes later. Listen to a type of music that's new to you. Rearrange your kitchen cabinets so that you have to think about where to find things. Overall, don't let your brain get into the rut of performing the same tasks over and over.

Fight Brain Inflammation

You've probably heard that good oral hygiene can reduce the risk for heart disease. A new study suggests that it also can promote brain health. Researchers found that men and women over age 60 who had the lowest levels of oral bacteria did better on cognitive tests involving memory and calculations than those who had more bacteria.

Why: Bacteria associated with gum disease also cause inflammation in the brain. This low-level inflammation can damage brain cells and affect cognitive function.

Simple thing you can do: Brush your teeth after every meal—and floss twice a day. I also recommend using an antiseptic mouthwash, which helps eliminate bacteria.

Getting Older Doesn't Have to Mean Getting Weaker

John E. Morley, MD, director of the division of geriatric medicine and the Dammert Professor of Gerontology at Saint Louis University School of Medicine. He is coeditor of the textbook *Sarcopenia* and editor of the professional publication *Journal of the American Medical Directors Association.* Dr. Morley is also a recipient of the American Geriatrics Society's Lascher/Manning Award for Lifetime Achievement in Geriatrics.

If you're age 50 or older, you've probably noticed that your suitcases and grocery bags have gotten mysteriously heavier. It's hard to admit it, but your muscle power is not what it used to be.

Unfortunately, far too many people assume that this age-related condition known as sarcopenia, which literally means "loss of muscle or flesh," is an inevitable part of aging. But that's simply not true. New and better ways to prevent and diagnose this condition now are available—and there's more reason than ever to not ignore it.

The dangers of sarcopenia are more serious than experts once thought—and may involve other crucial elements of your health such as your risk for diabetes, dementia and other chronic conditions.

More Than Muscle Loss

With advancing age, our muscles shrink because the body loses some of its ability to convert protein into muscle tissue. By age 50, the average adult loses about 1% to 2% of muscle mass every year.

That's bad enough, but the real problem is what results from this muscle loss. Over time, it becomes more difficult to stand up from a chair...climb a flight of stairs...or even open a jar. People with sarcopenia are far more likely than stronger adults to suffer falls and/or bone fractures. They're also more likely to be hospitalized or admitted to a nursing home—and even die during a given period of time.

An increasing body of evidence shows that people with weak muscle strength have a higher risk of developing type 2 diabetes—a disease that can also double your risk for heart attack and stroke.

Recently discovered danger: People with sarcopenia are at increased risk for cognitive decline, including brain atrophy and dementia, according to research published in *Clinical Interventions in Aging*. In this study, people with sarcopenia were six times more likely to suffer from physical/cognitive impairments than those without this condition.

What this means to you: Collectively, the risks associated with sarcopenia are so great that clinicians from a variety of disciplines assess signs such as weight loss (from shrinking muscles)...fatigue...and a loss of strength to determine which patients are at highest risk for frailty and to work toward intervention.

The Four-Step Plan

As scientists learn more about sarcopenia, the better your odds are of fighting it—if you take the appropriate steps. *What works best if you have sarcopenia...*

STEP 1: **Load up on protein.** Everyone needs protein to increase muscle size/strength. People with sarcopenia need a lot of protein. The recommended daily allowance (RDA) for protein is 0.8 g per kilogram of body weight. (That's about 54 g for a 150-pound woman.) If you've been diagnosed with sarcopenia, you need much more (about 1.2 g per kilogram of body weight).

My advice: Whenever possible, get most or all of your protein from natural foods rather than from protein-fortified foods—the nutrients in natural foods work synergistically to provide greater benefits than supplements. (For example, a small, 3.5-ounce serving of lean pork has about 26 g of protein… one-half cup of pinto beans, 7 g…and a large egg, about 6 g.)

Note: If you have kidney disease, you may have been told to limit your protein intake. Ask your nephrologist for advice on optimal protein levels for you.

Helpful: If you find it difficult to get enough protein from food alone, try whey protein supplements. You can buy these milk-based supplements in powder and liquid forms. Products such as Ensure typically provide 12 g to 20 g of protein per serving, while some protein powders deliver up to 60 g in two scoops mixed in a smoothie, for example. An advantage of whey protein supplements is that they contain leucine, an amino acid involved in muscle synthesis. If you can't have dairy, ask your doctor about taking an essential amino acid supplement enriched with leucine.

STEP 2: Get enough vitamin D. You need vitamin D for both muscle and bone strength. Depending upon the time of year and where you live, you can get all you need from 10 or so minutes of daily unprotected sun exposure. But many older adults don't spend that much time in the sun… and those who do are probably covering up or using sunscreen to protect against skin cancer.

My advice: Consume at least 1,000 international units (IU) of vitamin D daily. You can get some of this from D-fortified cereal, milk or juice. If you don't eat a lot of these foods, you may find it easier to take a 1,000-IU vitamin D supplement.

STEP 3: Eat fish. There's good evidence that two to four weekly meals of fatty fish (such as salmon, mackerel or sardines) will improve blood flow to all of the body's muscles, including the heart. In theory, this should help people with sarcopenia maintain or gain muscle mass, but the evidence that it helps isn't conclusive. Even so, I still recommend fish because it's a good protein source and has many other health benefits.

STEP 4: Exercise the right way. Exercise is the only way to build muscle, even if you consume plenty of protein. Aerobic exercise (such as brisk walking) is good—everyone should get some because it improves both muscle and cardiovascular health. But strength training is the real ticket for building muscle. As an added bonus, it also appears to promote brain health.

Important new finding: When Australian researchers had 100 people age 55 or older with mild cognitive impairment (a condition that often precedes Alzheimer's) do weight-lifting exercises twice a week for six months, the stronger the study participants' muscles got, the greater their cognitive improvement, according to a study published in 2016 in *Journal of the American Geriatrics Society.*

Even if you are not able to use weight-lifting machines at a gym, there are plenty of ways to do strength training. The American College of Sports Medicine recommends lifting weights (hand weights are fine) or using elastic resistance bands two to three days a week. Unfortunately, that's too ambitious for many people.

My advice: Just do some exercise, whether it's 10 minutes every day or an hour once a week. If you feel too weak to start with "real" exercise, you can keep things simple. Example: A chair-stand exercise, in which you sit in an armless chair...extend your arms in front of you...slowly stand up...then slowly lower yourself back down. Do this five to 10 times, twice daily.

For arm strength: Hold the ends of a large elastic resistance band in each hand, and stand with both feet on the middle of the band. Keeping your body straight and your elbows by your side, slowly curl your hands up toward your shoulders. You can raise both hands together or one at a time. Try to repeat the movement eight to 12 times, twice daily.

For leg strength: Sit on a chair. Keeping your back straight, slowly extend your right leg straight out in front of you and hold for several seconds before lowering it slowly back down. Repeat with the left leg. Do 10 repetitions on each leg. When this becomes easy, strap on an ankle weight that's heavy enough so that you cannot do more than 15 repetitions per leg.

If you tend to get bored with exercise, here's a great solution...

Research shows that people who work with an exercise coach or personal trainer—at home or at a health club—are more likely to stick with regular exercise. In a program that my colleagues and I supervise, patients with sarcopenia first attend physical therapy to help restore flexibility, balance and endurance, then attend weekly sessions led by exercise coaches who are enthusiastic and keep people motivated.

My advice: Consider using an exercise coach. It may be one of the best things you can do for your overall health! To find an exercise coach near you, consult the American Council on Exercise, ACEfitness.org.

The Three Supplements Everyone Should Take

Alan R. Gaby, MD, the contributing medical editor for *Townsend Letter*, contributing editor for *Alternative Medicine Review*, chief science editor for *Aisle 7* and the author of numerous scientific papers on nutritional medicine. His most recent book is the comprehensive textbook *Nutritional Medicine*, widely used by natural practitioners as a reference manual. DoctorGaby.com

I n an ideal world, we'd get all our nutrients from foods—there's a powerful synergistic effect when vitamins and minerals are found in foods. But the reality is, most people don't get enough of these crucial nutrients. That's why certain individual supplements can help.

In addition to an over-the-counter multivitamin, such as Centrum or One A Day, you may benefit from the following supplements because most multis don't contain enough of these nutrients.

Exception: If you use a high-potency multivitamin (it has megadoses of nutrients and is usually labeled "high potency"), you're most likely getting enough of the necessary nutrients and probably don't need to add the supplements below. But you may still need these additional supplements if you have any of the health conditions described in this article.

Three Key Supplements

Supplements everyone should consider taking...*

●**B-complex.** The B vitamins—thiamine, riboflavin, niacin and several others—are a must for the body's production of energy. They also play a key role in the health of the brain and nervous system.

But when foods are refined—for example, when kernels of whole wheat are stripped of their outer covering of fibrous bran and inner core of wheat germ and turned into white flour, as commonly occurs in American manufacturing practices—B vitamins are lost.

*Be sure to check with a nutrition-savvy health practitioner before taking any supplements. To find one near you, consult the Academy of Integrative Health and Medicine, AIHM.org, or the American Association of Naturopathic Physicians, Naturopathic.org.

Recent scientific evidence: A study of 104 middle-aged and older adults, published this summer, showed that taking three B vitamins (folic acid, B-6 and B-12) lowered levels of the amino acid homocysteine in people with very high levels (such elevations are linked to heart disease) and improved several measurements of mental functioning, such as memory.

Typical dose of B vitamins: Look for a B-complex supplement that contains at least 20 mg of most of the B vitamins, including B-6, thiamine and niacin…and at least 50 micrograms (mcg) each of B-12 and biotin.

•**Magnesium.** Without this mineral, your body couldn't produce energy, build bones, regulate blood sugar or even move a muscle. But most Americans don't get enough of this mineral in their diets.

Magnesium is used by nutritionally oriented clinicians to treat many health problems, including insomnia, chronic muscle pain, headache, heart disease, diabetes, osteoporosis and hearing loss. Overall, magnesium is the most beneficial supplement I have seen in my patients.

Typical dose of magnesium: 200 mg, twice a day. A capsule or a chewable or liquid form is preferable to a tablet, because it is more easily absorbed. But all types of magnesium—including magnesium oxide, magnesium citrate and magnesium aspartate—are equally effective for most conditions. If you develop diarrhea, reduce the dose until diarrhea eases.

•**Vitamin C.** This vitamin is an antioxidant—a nutrient that protects you from oxidation, a kind of inner rust that destroys cells. A low level of oxidation is normal, but it's increased by many factors—such as stress and chronic disease.

Recent finding: A review of 13 studies involving nearly 4,000 people with colorectal adenoma (a benign tumor that can turn into colon cancer) found that people with the highest levels of vitamin C were 22% less likely to develop colon cancer.

Typical dose of vitamin C: 100 mg to 500 mg daily, for general nutritional support. If you have a family history of colon cancer (for example, in a first-degree relative, such as a parent or sibling), consider taking 1,000 mg, three times daily.

"Add-On" Supplements You May Need

Certain people may need additional supplements to protect or improve their health. *Two key "add-on" supplements…*

•**Fish oil.** A large body of scientific research shows that fish oil can help prevent and treat heart disease.

Typical dose: About 1 g daily for people who want to reduce heart disease risk…and 2 g to 6 g daily for people diagnosed with the condition. People with coronary heart disease need 360 mg to 1,080 mg daily of eicosapentaenoic acid (EPA) and 240 mg to 720 mg of docosahexaenoic acid (DHA). Talk to a health practitioner before taking fish oil—it may increase bleeding risk.

•**Vitamin D.** Vitamin D deficiency is common, and it can increase risk for bone loss (osteoporosis), falls in older people (frailty), the flu, autoimmune diseases (such as rheumatoid arthritis, lupus and multiple sclerosis) and even cancer.

New thinking: 400 international units (IU) daily was once thought to preserve bone and prevent falls, but studies now show that 800 IU daily is preferable. Ask your doctor for advice on the best dose for you, and use vitamin D-3 (the type derived from sunlight and animal sources).

Five DIY Tests That Could Save Your Life

David L. Katz, MD, MPH, an internist and preventive medicine specialist. He is cofounder and director of the Yale-Griffin Prevention Research Center in Derby, Connecticut, and clinical instructor at the Yale School of Medicine in New Haven, Connecticut. Dr. Katz is also president of the American College of Lifestyle Medicine and the author of *Disease-Proof: The Remarkable Truth About What Makes Us Well.*

I f you're conscientious about your health, you probably see your doctor for an annual physical…or perhaps even more often if you have a chronic condition or get sick.

But if you'd like to keep tabs on your health between your doctor visits, there are some easy, do-it-yourself tests that can give you valuable information about your body. These tests can sometimes tip you off that you may have a serious medical condition even though you don't have any symptoms.

Here are self-tests that you can do at home—repeat them once every few months, and keep track of results. *See your doctor if you don't "pass" one or more of the tests…* *

Test #1: Stairs Test

Why this test? It helps assess basic lung and heart function.

*These self-tests are not a substitute for a thorough physical exam from your doctor. Use them only as a way to identify potential problem areas to discuss with your physician.

The prop you'll need: A single flight of stairs (about eight to 12 steps).

What to do: Walk up the steps at a normal pace while continuously reciting "Mary had a little lamb" or some other simple verse.

Watch out: You should be able to talk easily while climbing the stairs and when at the top—without feeling winded. If you cannot continue to talk, or if you feel discomfort or tightness in your chest at any time during this test, see your doctor as soon as possible.

Beware: If the small stress of climbing one flight of stairs causes physical problems, it could be a sign of hardening of the arteries (arteriosclerosis) or heart disease.

For some individuals, being out of breath could mean that they have asthma or bronchitis...chronic obstructive pulmonary disease (COPD), including emphysema...or even lung cancer.

Test #2: Gravity Test

Why this test? It measures how well your body adapts to changes in position, which can signal a variety of health problems, ranging from anemia to medication side effects.

The prop you'll need: Either a stopwatch or clock that measures seconds.

What to do: Lie down on a bed or the floor, and rest there for a minute or two. Then, start the stopwatch and stand up at a normal pace with no pauses (it's OK to use your hands).

Watch out: If you feel dizzy, make note of this. Most people can go from lying down to standing up within five seconds—and feel perfectly normal. In a healthy person, the body responds to the change in posture by pumping blood more strongly to the head.

Beware: Dizziness can signal any of the following...

•**Low blood pressure.**

With *orthostatic hypotension,* your body doesn't pump enough blood to counteract the effects of gravity when you stand up.

•**Medication side effects,** especially from diuretics, such as *furosemide* (Lasix)...beta-blockers, such as *atenolol* (Tenormin) or *propranolol* (Inderal)... drugs for Parkinson's disease, such as *pramipexole* (Mirapex) or *levodopa* (Sinemet)...tricyclic antidepressants, such as *imipramine* (Tofranil) or *amitriptyline* (Elavil)...or drugs to treat erectile dysfunction, such as *sildenafil* (Viagra) or *tadalafil* (Cialis).

- **Dehydration.**
- **Anemia.**
- **Atherosclerosis,** in which blood flow is partially blocked by fatty deposits in blood vessels, or other vascular problems.

Test #3: Pencil Test

Why this test? It checks the nerve function in your feet—if abnormal, this could indicate diabetes, certain types of infections or autoimmune disease.

The prop you'll need: A pencil that is freshly sharpened at one end with a flat eraser on the other end…and a friend to help.

What to do: Sit down so that all sides of your bare feet are accessible. Close your eyes, and keep them closed throughout the test.

Have your friend lightly touch your foot with either the sharp end or the eraser end of the pencil. With each touch, say which end of the pencil you think was used.

Ask your friend to repeat the test in at least three different locations on the tops and bottoms of both feet (12 locations total). Have your friend keep track of your right and wrong answers.

Watch out: Most people can easily tell the difference between "sharp" and "dull" sensations on their sensitive feet. If you give the wrong answer for more than two or three locations on your feet, have your doctor repeat the test to determine whether you have nerve damage (neuropathy).

Beware: Neuropathy is a common sign of diabetes…certain autoimmune disorders, including lupus and Sjögren's syndrome…infection, such as Lyme disease, shingles or hepatitis C…or excessive exposure to toxins, such as pesticides or heavy metals (mercury or lead).

Test #4: Urine Test

Why this test? It helps evaluate the functioning of your kidneys.

The prop you'll need: A clear plastic cup or clean, disposable clear jar.

What to do: In the middle of the day (urine will be too concentrated if you do this first thing in the morning), urinate into the cup or jar until you have caught at least an inch of urine. Throughout the day, note how often you urinate (about once every three waking hours is typical).

Watch out: The urine should be a pale, straw color—not deep yellow, brown or pinkish. Urine that's discolored could indicate dehydration, abnormal kidney function or another health problem.

Next, smell the urine. It should have nothing more than a very faint urine odor (unless you recently ate asparagus).

Beware: While dark-colored or smelly urine could simply mean that you are dehydrated, there are too many other potentially serious causes to ignore the signs.

Some of the disorders that can affect urine include...

•**Kidney or bladder infection,** which can cause discolored urine and frequent urination.

•**Kidney disease,** which can cause smelly, discolored urine. Interestingly, both too frequent urination and infrequent urination are signs of kidney disease.

•**Diabetes or enlarged prostate,** which can cause frequent urination.

Test #5: "Rule of Thumb" Test

Why this test? It can help identify hearing loss.

The prop you'll need: A perfectly quiet room.

What to do: Rub your right thumb and index finger together continuously to create a kind of "whisper" sound. Raise your right arm so that it's level with your ear and your arm is roughly forming a right angle. Continue rubbing your thumb and index finger together. Can you still hear the sound? If not, move your hand toward your right ear, stopping when you can just hear the sound. Repeat on the left side.

Watch out: You should be able to hear this "finger rub" when your hand is six inches or more away from your ear.

Beware: If you need to be closer than six inches to hear the sound in either ear, you may have hearing loss. See an audiologist or otolaryngologist (ear, nose and throat specialist) for an evaluation.

While many people dismiss hearing loss as a mere inconvenience, it can have serious repercussions, such as getting into a car wreck because you can't hear the sound of a car approaching from the side.

CHAPTER 2

Eat Like This for Longevity

Five Surprising Foods to Help You Live Longer

Bonnie Taub-Dix, RD, a registered dietitian and owner of BTD Nutrition Consultants located in New York City. A nationally recognized nutrition expert and the author of *Read It Before You Eat It*, she has advised patients on the best ways to control diabetes for more than three decades. BonnieTaubDix.com

Whether your blood sugar (glucose) levels are normal and you want to keep them that way…or you have diabetes and glucose control is your mantra…it is smart to eat a well-balanced diet to help keep your glucose readings healthy. In fact, maintaining healthy glucose levels may even help you live longer by avoiding diabetes—one of the leading causes of death in the US.

Most people already know that cinnamon is an excellent choice for blood sugar control. Consuming just one-half teaspoon to three teaspoons a day can reduce glucose levels by up to 24%. Cinnamon is great on cereals, vegetables, cottage cheese and snacks (think fresh apple slices sprinkled with cinnamon).

Other smart food choices…*

Glucose-Controlling Food #1: BLACK BEANS

Beans, in general, are the most underrated food in the supermarket.

Beans are high in protein as well as soluble and insoluble fiber. Soluble fiber helps you feel fuller longer, and insoluble fiber helps prevent constipa-

*If you take diabetes medication, consult your doctor before making significant changes to your diet—drug dosages may need to be adjusted.

tion. Beans also break down slowly during digestion, which means more stable blood sugar levels.

Black beans, however, are particularly healthful because of their especially high fiber content. For example, one cup of cooked black beans contains 15 g of fiber, while a cup of pink beans has just 9 g.

Bonus: Beans protect the heart by lowering cholesterol and reducing damage from free radicals. For example, one study showed that you can lower your total and LDL ("bad") cholesterol by about 8% simply by eating one-half cup of cooked pinto beans every day.

Helpful: To shorten cooking times, use canned beans instead of dried beans. They are equally nutritious, and you can reduce the sodium in salted canned beans by about 40% by rinsing them.

Another healthful way to use beans: Hummus. In the Middle East, people eat this chickpea (garbanzo bean) spread as often as Americans eat bread. It is much healthier than bread because it contains both protein and olive oil—important for slowing the absorption of carbohydrate sugars and preventing blood sugar "spikes."

Hummus is a good weight-loss dish because it is high in fiber (about 15 g per cup) as well as protein (about 19 g). Ample amounts of protein and fiber allow you to satisfy your appetite with smaller portions of food.

Hummus is made with mashed chickpeas, tahini (a sesame seed paste), lemon juice, garlic, salt and a little olive oil. Stick to the serving size on the label, which is typically two to four tablespoons.

Glucose-Controlling Food #2: COCOA

The flavanols in cocoa are potent antioxidants that not only fight heart disease but also help guard against diabetes. In recent studies, cocoa improved insulin sensitivity, the body's ability to transport sugar out of the bloodstream. It's wise for people with diabetes or high blood sugar to choose unsweetened cocoa and add a small amount of sugar or sugar substitute.

Cinnamon hot cocoa combines two glucose-controlling ingredients in one delicious recipe.

To prepare: Mix one-quarter cup of baking cocoa, one tablespoon of sugar (or Truvia to taste) and a pinch of salt. Gradually add one-quarter cup of boiling water and blend well. Add one cup of skim or 1% low-fat milk and a cinnamon stick. While stirring occasionally, heat on low for 10 minutes. Remove the cinnamon stick and enjoy!

Glucose-Controlling Food #3: DATES

These little fruits are sweet enough to qualify as dessert but have more anti-oxidants per serving than oranges, grapes and even broccoli. The antioxidants can help prevent heart disease as well as neuropathy—nerve damage that frequently occurs in people who have diabetes.

A single serving (for example, seven deglet noor dates) has 4 g of fiber for better blood sugar management.

Be careful: Seven dates also have 140 calories and 32 g of sugar, so this must be added to your total daily carbohydrate intake, especially if you have diabetes. Dates, in general, have a low glycemic index, so they don't spike glucose levels. Medjool dates, however, are not an ideal choice. They have significantly more sugar and calories per serving than deglet noor dates.

Glucose-Controlling Food #4: SARDINES

Many people know about the heart-healthy benefits of cold-water fish, such as salmon and mackerel. An analysis of studies involving hundreds of thousands of adults found that just one to two fish servings a week reduced the risk of dying from heart disease by more than one-third.

What's less well known is that the high concentration of omega-3 fatty acids in cold-water fish also helps prevent a too-rapid rise in blood sugar. Besides being low on the glycemic index, fish contains protein, which blunts blood sugar levels.

Best for helping to prevent high blood sugar: In addition to salmon and mackerel, sardines are an excellent choice (when canned with bones, they also are a good source of calcium). Tuna, to a somewhat lesser extent, offers omega-3s (choose canned light—albacore white has higher levels of mercury). Also avoid large fish, such as king mackerel and swordfish, which have more mercury than smaller fish. Aim for a 3.5-ounce serving two or three times a week.

Glucose-Controlling Food #5: ALMONDS

High in fiber, protein and beneficial fats, nuts can significantly lower glucose levels. In fact, women who ate a one-ounce serving of nuts at least five times a week were nearly 30% less likely to develop diabetes than women who rarely or never ate nuts, according to one study.

The poly- and monounsaturated fats in nuts improve the body's ability to use insulin. Nuts also help with cholesterol control—important because diabetes increases risk for heart disease.

All nuts are beneficial, but almonds contain more fiber, calcium and protein than most nuts (and are best for blood sugar control). Walnuts are highest in antioxidants and omega-3 fatty acids. Avoid salted nuts—they have too much sodium.

Excellent way to add nuts to your diet: Nut butters. Almost everyone likes peanut butter, and it is healthier than you might think. Like butters made from almonds, cashews or other nuts, the fats it contains are mostly monounsaturated, which are good for the heart. The fiber in nut butters (about 1 g to 2 g per tablespoon, depending on the nut) can help lower blood sugar.

Good choice for blood sugar control: One serving (one to two tablespoons) of almond butter (rich in potassium, vitamin E and calcium) several times a week. Look for nut butters that have a short list of ingredients—they are the most nutritious.

A Simple Blood Sugar Buster

Taking two tablespoons of apple-cider vinegar in eight ounces of water with meals or before bedtime can slow the absorption of sugar into the blood—vinegar helps to block the digestive enzymes that change carbs to sugar.

Eat Your Way to Health: DASH Diet

Marla Heller, MS, RD, author of *The DASH Diet Action Plan,* based in Chicago. Her website is DASHDiet.org/Marla.asp.

Maintaining normal blood pressure is vital to staying healthy, but perhaps we've been trained by the mainstream medical community to rely too much on drugs to do it. For many people, there can be a better—and safer—way that requires nothing more than your spoon and fork.

During a five-center study in the 1990s sponsored by the National Institutes of Health, researchers found that participants with high blood pressure (hypertension) who followed a specific dietary plan called DASH (Dietary Approaches to Stop Hypertension) lowered systolic pressure (the higher number in a blood pressure reading) by 11.4 mm/Hg and diastolic pressure by 6 mm/Hg. More recent studies gave the DASH diet added value—at Brigham and

Women's Hospital in Boston, an analysis of data from the long-term Nurse's Health Study and Health Professionals Follow-Up Study found that following the DASH diet was associated with lower risk for kidney stones. Other studies find that a DASH diet lowers risk for cardiac disease and stroke…and most recently, at Utah State University in Logan, an 11-year study has demonstrated that elderly adults who followed DASH stayed mentally sharp longer.

How to Do DASH

The diet (more details to follow) basically consists of eating healthy foods with some specific tweaking, plus a salt limitation. Given that the typical diet of Americans today is filled with processed foods high in sugar, salt and fat, DASH is often described as "difficult to follow." But it doesn't have to be! It usually takes time to overcome a lifetime of bad habits such as living on french fries and soft drinks…but the DASH plan includes a wide variety of delicious, satisfying foods. It is important to follow this dietary plan closely because in addition to restricting sodium, eating the recommended amounts of foods on DASH provides high amounts of magnesium, potassium and calcium. A diet that is rich in foods with this combination of nutrients is what helps to control blood pressure.

In a nutshell, here's the DASH diet…

•**Whole grains**—six to eight servings a day of products made from 100% whole grains…a serving is one slice of bread, one ounce of dry cereal, or one-half cup of cooked cereal, whole-grain pasta or brown rice.

•**Fruits and vegetables**—eight to 10 servings a day…a serving is defined as one cup of raw, leafy vegetables or one-half cup of cooked veggies, one medium fruit, one-half cup low-sodium vegetable juice, one cup of fresh fruit, or one-half cup of frozen or canned fruit. To reduce calories, you should limit starchy vegetables, such as potatoes, corn and the like, but the good news is that you can eat as much as you like of the nonstarchy ones, for example, tomatoes, green beans, leafy greens, peppers and others.

•**Low-fat or nonfat dairy**—two to three servings a day. A serving is one cup of milk or yogurt or one and one-half ounces of cheese.

•**Lean meat, fish and poultry**—six or fewer ounces a day. A three-ounce serving is the size of a pack of cards, which is sufficient with a meal.

•**Nuts, seeds and beans**—four to five servings per week…servings include one-half cup of cooked dried beans or peas, one-quarter cup of nuts or two tablespoons of peanut butter. It is okay to have more beans than this each week, but if so you should balance that by eating less meat, fish and poultry.

• **Fats and oils**—two to three servings a day...with a serving being one teaspoon of margarine or vegetable oil, one tablespoon of mayonnaise or two tablespoons of salad dressing.

• **Sweets**—up to five servings a week...such as one-half cup sorbet, one tablespoon of sugar, jelly or jam, or one cup of lemonade.

• **Sodium**—The National Academy of Science's Institute of Medicine recommends not exceeding 1,500 mg to 2,400 mg of salt per day (1,500 mg is about two-thirds teaspoon of table salt).

Note: Factors such as medications you are on, exercise and diet history should be considered in determining your optimal sodium intake.

Make DASH Delicious...

Here's another reason the DASH diet is tastier and easier to follow than you might think: It follows many of the same principles as the Mediterranean Diet that is so popular today, in particular its focus on a daily bounty of fresh vegetables. It's easy to find restaurants serving these foods.

While many new DASH followers complain about a lack of flavor, what they really are reacting to is the lack of salt. Here are some favorite cooking tips for flavorful food—and note that reducing salt intake is easier if you make the change gradually. Try using a base of onions, garlic and red wine, which makes just about everything tasty. For sautéing foods, I start with onions and garlic together and at the very end of the dish I add a little bit of red wine and cook it down to evaporate the alcohol. Herbs add flavor, too—for instance, try a bit of oregano or thyme on vegetables. A sprinkle of reduced-sodium cheese can also be delicious, as is, surprisingly, cinnamon. Another trick is to drizzle a bit of olive oil (a tablespoon) over foods, which enhances their flavor and adds fat, making them more satisfying and also helping with absorption of nutrients.

To get started on DASH, it is vital to clear your kitchen and pantry of all foods that are not on the diet. Then stock up with a wide variety of fresh, tasty and healthy DASH foods. That way, when your stomach rumbles, you will have plenty of satisfying no-cheat choices. For more information on DASH, suggested menus and recipes, go to DashDiet.org.

Foods That Sabotage Sleep

Bonnie Taub-Dix, RD, a registered dietitian and owner of BTD Nutrition Consultants located in New York City. A nationally recognized nutrition expert and the author of *Read It Before You Eat It*, she has advised patients on the best ways to control diabetes for more than three decades. BonnieTaubDix.com

You know that an evening coffee can leave you tossing and turning in the wee hours. But other foods hurt sleep, too…

●**Premium ice cream.** Brace yourself for a restless night if you indulge in Häagen-Dazs or Ben & Jerry's late at night. The richness of these wonderful treats comes mainly from fat—16 to 17 grams (g) of fat in half a cup of vanilla and who eats just half a cup?

Your body digests fat more slowly than it digests proteins or carbohydrates. When you eat a high-fat food within an hour or two of bedtime, your digestion will still be "active" when you lie down—and that can disturb sleep.

Also, the combination of stomach acid, stomach contractions and a horizontal position increases the risk for reflux, the upsurge of digestive juices into the esophagus that causes heartburn—which can disturb sleep.

●**Chocolate.** Some types of chocolate can jolt you awake almost as much as a cup of coffee. Dark chocolate, in particular, has shocking amounts of caffeine.

Example: Half a bar of Dagoba Eclipse Extra Dark has 41 milligrams of caffeine, close to what you'd get in a shot of mild espresso.

Chocolate also contains theobromine, another stimulant, which is never a good choice near bedtime.

●**Beans.** Beans are one of the healthiest foods. But a helping or two of beans—or broccoli, cauliflower, cabbage or other gas-producing foods—close to bedtime can make your night, well, a little noisier than usual. No one sleeps well when suffering from gas pains. You can reduce the "backtalk" by drinking a mug of chamomile or peppermint tea at bedtime. They're carminative herbs that aid digestion and help prevent gas.

Fiber Helps You Live Longer

In a recent study, researchers followed more than 388,000 volunteers, ages 50 to 71, and found that men and women who consumed the most fiber were 24% to 59% less likely to die from infections, heart disease or respiratory illness than those who did not.

Possible reason: Fiber may steady blood sugar, lower blood lipids and control inflammation.

Recommended: 21 to 25 grams of fiber daily for women and 30 to 38 grams for men from naturally occurring plant-based sources, such as grains, legumes, vegetables and fruits. Commercially made foods that are fortified with fiber were not studied.

Yikyung Park, ScD, staff scientist, National Cancer Institute, Bethesda, Maryland, and leader of a study of more than 388,000 people, published in *Archives of Internal Medicine.*

•**Spicy foods.** Spicy foods temporarily speed up your metabolism. They are associated with taking longer to fall asleep and with more time spent awake at night. This may be caused by the capsaicin found in chile peppers, which affect body temperature and disrupt sleep. Also, in some people, spicy foods can lead to sleep-disturbing gas, stomach cramps and heartburn.

Foods That Help You Sleep

Carbohydrate-based meals increase blood levels of tryptophan, used by the body to manufacture serotonin, a "calming" neurotransmitter. *Also helpful…*

•**Warm milk.** It's not a myth—warm milk at bedtime really will help you get to sleep. It settles the stomach, and the ritual of drinking it can help you calm down and fall asleep more easily.

•**Cherry juice.** A study published in *Journal of Medicinal Food* found that people who drank eight ounces of tart cherry juice in the morning and eight at night for two weeks had about 17 minutes less awake time during the night than when they drank a non-cherry juice. Tart cherries are high in melatonin, a hormone that regulates the body's sleep-wake cycles. The brand used in the study was Cheribundi.

Helpful: Tart cherry juice has 140 calories in eight ounces, so you may want to cut back on calories elsewhere.

Got This? Don't Eat That

Michael T. Murray, ND, a naturopathic physician and leading authority on natural medicine. Dr. Murray serves on the Board of Regents of Bastyr University in Kenmore, Washington, and has written more than 30 books, including *The Encyclopedia of Natural Medicine* with coauthor Joseph Pizzorno, ND. DoctorMurray.com

Let's say you've got arthritis…heartburn…heart disease…or some other common health problem.

You follow all your doctor's suggestions, but you still don't feel better. It could be that you're not getting the right medication or other treatment, but there's an even stronger possibility.

What often gets overlooked: Your diet. Far too many people sabotage their treatment—and actually make their health problems worse—by eating the wrong foods. Meanwhile, you could be helping yourself by eating certain foods that ease whatever is ailing you.

Common health problems that foods can worsen—or help...

Arthritis

Both osteoarthritis and rheumatoid arthritis involve inflammation that causes joint pain and/or swelling.

What hurts: Refined carbohydrates (sugar, white bread, white rice and most pasta). They cause a spike in glucose (blood sugar) that leads to inflammation.

What helps: Raw, fresh ginger. It's a potent inhibitor of prostaglandin and thromboxanes, inflammatory compounds involved in arthritis. And unlike anti-inflammatory medications, ginger doesn't cause an upset stomach. Be sure to use fresh ginger—it's better than powdered because it contains higher levels of active ingredients. For pain relief, you need to eat only about 10 g (about a quarter-inch slice) of raw, fresh ginger a day.

Smart idea: You can add raw ginger to any fresh fruit or vegetable juice with the help of a juice extractor. Ginger mixes well with carrot, apple, pear or pineapple juice. You also can grate fresh ginger and add it to any hot tea.

Cardiac Arrhythmias

Everyone notices occasional changes in the way the heart beats at certain times—during exercise, for example. But persistent irregularities could be a sign of arrhythmias, potentially dangerous problems with the heart's electrical system. The heart can skip beats or beat too slowly or too quickly—all of which can signal heart disease.

What hurts: Too much caffeine. Whether it's in coffee, tea or chocolate, caffeine stimulates the heart to beat more quickly, which triggers arrhythmias in some people.

What helps: Berries. All types of berries, including cherries, blackberries, raspberries and blueberries, are rich in procyanidins, plant pigments that reduce arrhythmias and improve blood flow through the coronary arteries. Aim for one cup of fresh berries daily (frozen are fine, too).

Also helpful: Concentrated extracts made from hawthorn. This herb contains the same heart-healthy compounds as berries. In Germany, it is commonly used to treat arrhythmias and congestive heart failure. If you have heart problems, a hawthorn extract containing 10% procyanidins (100 mg to 200 mg three times daily) is often recommended. Hawthorn can interact with heart medications and other drugs, so check with your doctor before trying it.

Heartburn

Also known as gastroesophageal reflux disease (GERD), heartburn is usually caused by the upward surge of digestive juices from the stomach into the esophagus. People who suffer from frequent heartburn can get some relief with lifestyle changes, such as not overeating and staying upright for a few hours after eating. But most people with heartburn don't pay enough attention to their diets.

What hurts: Alcohol and coffee are widely known to trigger heartburn. Many people, however, don't consider the effects of chocolate, fried foods and carbonated drinks, which also may weaken the esophageal sphincter (the muscle that prevents acids from entering the esophagus) or increase the intra-abdominal pressure that pushes acids upward.

What helps: Fresh (not bottled) lemon juice—two to four ounces daily in water, tea or apple or carrot juices. Lemon contains D-limonene, an oil-based compound that helps prevent heartburn. Also, use the peel if you can. It's an especially good source of D-limonene.

Eye Disease

Age-related macular degeneration (AMD) is a leading cause of vision loss, but it (as well as cataracts) can often be prevented—or the effects—by eating carefully.

What hurts: Animal fat and processed foods. A study of 261 adults with AMD found that people who ate a lot of these foods were twice as likely to have a worsening of their eye disease compared with those who ate less of the foods. Animal fat also increases risk for high cholesterol, which has been linked to increased risk for cataracts.

What helps: Cold-water fish. The omega-3 fatty acids in fish can help prevent AMD and cataracts—or, if you already have one of these conditions, help prevent it from getting worse. Try to eat three to four weekly servings of cold-water fish, such as salmon or sardines.

Also helpful: Tomatoes, watermelon and other red fruits and vegetables (such as red peppers) that are high in lycopene. Green vegetables are also protective. Foods such as spinach and kale are high in lutein and other plant pigments that concentrate in the retina to help prevent eye disease.

Rosacea

Some 16 million Americans have rosacea, a chronic skin condition that causes bright-red facial flushing for at least 10 minutes per episode, along with bumps and pustules.

What hurts: Hot foods. "Hot" can mean temperature (a hot bowl of soup or a steaming cup of coffee or tea) or spicy (such as chili powder, cayenne or curry). Alcohol also tends to increase flushes.

What helps: If you have rosacea, ask your doctor to test you for H. pylori, the bacterium that causes most stomach ulcers and has been linked to rosacea. If you test positive, drink cabbage juice (eight to 12 ounces daily). It's not the tastiest juice, but it inhibits the growth of H. pylori. Make your own cabbage juice in a juicer (add some apples and/or carrots to improve the taste). If you have thyroid problems, check with your doctor—fresh cabbage may interfere with thyroid function.

Six Herbs That Slow Aging

Donald R. Yance, CN, MH, RH (AHG), clinical master herbalist and certified nutritionist. He is medical director at the Mederi Foundation's Centre for Natural Healing in Ashland, Oregon…founder and president of the Mederi Foundation, a not-for-profit organization for professional education and clinical research in collaborative medicine…and president and formulator of Natura Health Products. He is author of *Adaptogens in Medical Herbalism* and *Herbal Medicine, Healing & Cancer.* DonnieYance.com

You can't escape aging. But many Americans are aging prematurely.

Surprising fact: The US ranks 42nd out of 191 countries in life expectancy, according to the Census Bureau and the National Center for Health Statistics.

The leading cause of this rapid, premature aging is chronic stress. Stress is any factor, positive or negative, that requires the body to make a response or change to adapt. It can be psychological stress, including the modern addiction to nonstop stimulation and speed. Or it can be physiological stress—such as eating a highly processed diet…sitting for hours every day…absorbing toxins from food, water and air…and spending time in artificial light.

Chronic stress overwhelms the body's homeostasis, its inborn ability to adapt to stress and stay balanced, strong and healthy. The result?

Your hormonal and immune systems are weakened. Inflammation flares up, damaging cells. Daily energy decreases, fatigue increases, and you can't manage life as effectively. You suffer from one or more illnesses, take several medications and find yourself in a downward spiral of worsening health. Even though you might live to be 75 or older, you're surviving, not thriving.

We can reduce stress by making lifestyle changes such as eating better and exercising. You also can help beat stress and slow aging with adaptogens. These powerful herbs balance and strengthen the hormonal and immune systems...give you more energy...and repair cellular damage—thereby boosting your body's ability to adapt to chronic stress.

Important: Adaptogens are generally safe, but always talk with your doctor before taking any supplement.

Here are six of the most powerful adaptogens...

Ashwagandha

This adaptogen from Ayurveda (the ancient system of natural healing from India) can help with a wide range of conditions.

Main actions: It is energizing and improves sleep, and it can help with arthritis, anxiety, depression, dementia and respiratory disorders, such as asthma, bronchitis and emphysema.

Important benefit: It is uniquely useful for cancer—it can help kill cancer cells...reduce the toxicity of chemotherapy (and prevent resistance to chemotherapeutic drugs)...relieve cancer-caused fatigue...and prevent recurrence.

Eleuthero

This is the most well-researched adaptogen (with more than 3,000 published studies). It often is called the "king" of adaptogens. (It was introduced in the US as "Siberian ginseng," but it is not a ginseng.)

Main actions: Along with providing energy and vitality, eleuthero protects the body against the ill effects of any kind of stress, such as extremes of heat or cold, excessive exercise and radiation. More than any other adaptogen, it helps normalize any type of physiological abnormality—including high or low blood pressure...and high or low blood sugar.

Important benefit: Eleuthero is a superb "ergogenic" (performance-enhancing) aid that can help anyone involved in sports improve strength and endurance and recover from injury.

Ginseng

Used as a traditional medicine in Asia for more than 5,000 years and the subject of more than 500 scientific papers, ginseng has two primary species—*Panax ginseng* (Korean or Asian ginseng) and *Panax quinquefolius* (American ginseng).

Main actions: Ginseng is antifatigue and antiaging. It increases muscle strength and endurance and improves reaction times. It also strengthens the immune system and the heart and helps regulate blood sugar.

Important benefits: American ginseng can be beneficial for recovering from the common cold, pneumonia or bronchitis (particularly with a dry cough)...and chronic stress accompanied by depression or anxiety.

Korean or Asian ginseng is helpful for increasing physical performance, especially endurance and energy. It is effective for restoring adrenal function and neurological health such as learning and memory.

Rhaponticum

This herb contains more anabolic (strengthening and muscle-building) compounds than any other plant. It is my number-one favorite herb for increasing stamina and strength.

Main actions: It normalizes the central nervous and cardiovascular systems...improves sleep, appetite and mood...and increases the ability to work and function under stressful conditions.

Important benefit: This herb is wonderful for anyone recovering from injury, trauma or surgery.

Rhodiola

Rhodiola has gained popularity over the past few years as studies show that it rivals eleuthero and ginseng as an adaptogen. It is widely used by Russian athletes to increase energy.

Main actions: Rhodiola increases blood supply to the muscles and the brain, enhancing physical and mental performance, including memory. It normalizes the cardiovascular system and protects the heart from stress. It also strengthens immunity.

Red flag: Don't use rhodiola alone—it is extremely astringent and drying. It is best used along with other adaptogens in a formula.

Schisandra

This herb has a long history of use as an adaptogen in China, Russia, Japan, Korea and Tibet. The fruit is commonly used, but the seed is more powerful.

Main actions: Schisandra can treat stress-induced fatigue...protect and detoxify the liver...treat insomnia, depression and vision problems...and enhance athletic performance.

Important benefit: This adaptogen may help night vision—one study showed it improved adaptation to darkness by 90%.

Combinations Are Best

Any one herb has limitations in its healing power. But a combination or formula of adaptogenic herbs overcomes those limitations—because the adaptogens act in concert, making them more powerful.

This concept of synergy—multiple herbs acting together are more effective than one herb acting alone—is key to the effectiveness of the herbal formulas of traditional Chinese medicine (TCM) and Ayurveda. Both these ancient forms of medicine often employ a dozen or more herbs in their formulas.

But it's not only the combination of herbs that makes them effective—it's also the quality of the herbs. There are many more poor-quality adaptogens on the market than high-quality (or even mediocre-quality).

My advice: Look for an herbalist or herbal company that knows all about the source and content of the herbs it uses.

Example: Herbalist & Alchemist, a company that grows most of the herbs used in its products.

Or find a product sold to health practitioners, who then sell it to their patients—this type of product is more likely to be high quality.

Example: MediHerb, from Standard Process.

Herbal formulas from my company, Natura Health Products, also meet these criteria for high quality.

CHAPTER 3

Stay Fit for Longevity

Exercises That Help With Everything You Do

Larkin Barnett, an adjunct professor of exercise science at Florida Atlantic University in Boca Raton, and the author of *Functional Fitness: The Ultimate Fitness Program for Life on the Run.*

Functional training is a form of exercise that strengthens the muscles that we use in everyday activities, such as standing, walking, sitting, doing chores and carrying packages.

How it works: Functional training helps integrate the limbs and the trunk muscles for fluid, powerful movements...puts your body into proper alignment...improves posture and balance...and promotes deep breathing for relaxation.

A functional fitness routine can be incorporated into cardiovascular and strength-training workouts. *The exercises described below are designed for people of all fitness levels and should be performed daily...*

Sit Up and Take Notice

Benefits: Corrects trunk alignment, including weak abdominal muscles that don't provide sufficient support for the lower back...and enhances stamina and endurance.

Good for: Carrying objects...walking and running...and relieving muscle tension caused by working at a desk or a computer.

What to do: While sitting in a straight-backed chair, scrunch your shoulders up toward your ears, then relax them. Inhale slowly while you raise your shoulders, then exhale slowly as you lower them. Do this three to five times, feeling tension drain out of your shoulders and neck.

Next, sit tall, perched on your sit-bones (you can find these by rocking side-to-side) and concentrate on stacking your hips, ribs, chest and head on top of each other like building blocks. Exhale powerfully while pulling your abdominal muscles inward toward your spine. Then pull your shoulders back gently. Take several deep breaths.

Finally, sit up tall, while picturing the tops of your ears stretching upward. This elongates the spine and improves respiratory function. Tighten your abdominals inward and upward toward your spine while exhaling forcefully three to five times.

The Compass

Benefits: Strengthens your postural muscles (to improve coordination and balance)...and reduces fatigue and stress on the legs, hips and back.

Good for: Relieving muscle soreness from extended standing as well as improving performance in all sports and physical activities.

What to do: With your feet flat on the ground about 12 inches apart, pretend you're standing in the middle of a large compass. With exaggerated movements, shift your entire body toward each of the four main points on the compass—north (forward), south (backward), east (to the right) and west (to the left)—pausing momentarily at each point. Do this three to five times. Contract your abdominal muscles and notice how your control improves.

Gradually make your movements smaller and smaller. Do this for 30 seconds. End by standing still and feeling your body weight evenly distributed.

The Pelvis as a Fish Bowl

Benefits: Centers the hips and places the pelvis in neutral alignment, reducing stress on the legs, back and neck.

Good for: Lifting...getting in and out of bed...and swinging a golf club or tennis racket.

What to do: Standing with your feet about 12 inches apart, contract your stomach muscles and draw them inward and up toward your spine. Picture your hips as a fish bowl filled with water, with the bowl's rim at your waistline.

Now tip your hips forward slightly and visualize water spilling out of the front of the fish bowl. Next, tip your hips backward slightly and visualize water sloshing out of the back of the bowl. Finally, balance the fish bowl so that the rim is perfectly level. This is your pelvis's "neutral" position. Throughout the day, assume this position as you stand up, walk and sit.

Shoulder Blade, Arm, Fingertip

Benefits: Teaches you to initiate arm movements from your trunk muscles (including your shoulder girdle muscles) for more power and control.

Good for: Relieving muscle tension caused by driving a car or speaking on the telephone...and playing golf and racket sports.

What to do: While standing, lift your arms to your sides at shoulder level. Then lift your arms higher, in the shape of a "U," while sliding your shoulder blades downward. Imagine that you have a balloon next to each ear. Initiate these movements from the shoulder blades. Lower your arms, then repeat three to five times.

Which Exercises Are Best for You?

John P. Porcari, PhD, program director of the Clinical Exercise Physiology (CEP) program at the University of Wisconsin–La Crosse.

Everyone agrees that exercise is good for you. The goal for most people should be at least 150 minutes of moderate aerobic activity a week, plus strength training two days a week, according to the Centers for Disease Control and Prevention.

But what if you have a chronic condition, such as heart disease, arthritis, lung disease or Parkinson's disease, that makes exercise difficult—or raises your concern about injury?

While exercise is helpful for most chronic health problems, some activities are likely to be easier, more beneficial and less risky than others.* *Best workouts if you have...*

*Always talk to your doctor before starting a new exercise program. If you have a chronic illness, it may be useful to consult a physical therapist for advice on exercise dos and don'ts for your particular situation.

Cardiovascular Disease

A key benefit of exercise is reduced heart attack risk. But if you have already had a heart attack or undergone bypass surgery...or have symptoms, such as chest pain (angina), that signal established heart disease, you may worry that physical exertion is too risky.

For the vast majority of people with heart disease, it's not—if it's supervised. This usually involves initial and periodic testing to establish safe levels of exercise and monitoring of heart rate and blood pressure for some sessions. Once you're cleared, you can do most sessions on your own.

When performed at the proper intensity, standard aerobic activities are usually suitable. This means you can most likely walk, jog, use a stationary bike or treadmill (or even participate in aerobic dance) as long as you do it at a moderate level that doesn't raise your heart rate too high. Talk to your doctor about the heart rate you should strive for.

Once you have that number, you may want to wear a heart rate monitor—several models are widely available for under $100.

Another option: Use the "Talk Test." If you can talk while exercising, this will indicate with 95% accuracy that your heart rate is in a safe range.

If you have hypertension: Higher-intensity exercise may trigger potentially dangerous spikes in your blood pressure—talk to your doctor about appropriate heart rate goals, and remember to breathe (do not hold your breath) and stay away from heavier weights when doing strength training.

Important: Be sure to ask your doctor to reevaluate your target heart rate if you change blood pressure medication—some drugs, such as beta-blockers, will affect your heart rate.

Diabetes

Exercise can lower blood sugar almost as well as medication. Recent guidelines for people with diabetes recommend 150 minutes of moderate to strenuous aerobic exercise weekly, in addition to three strength-training sessions that work all the major muscle groups—increasing muscle mass is believed to be a particularly effective way of controlling blood sugar.

All aerobic exercises are beneficial, but those that use both your upper- and lower-body muscles are best because they help deliver blood glucose to muscle cells throughout your body—try an elliptical machine, the Schwinn Airdyne (a stationary bike that adds arm movements) or NuStep (a recumbent stepper that incorporates arm movements). If you walk, use poles to involve your arms. Try to do some type of exercise every day—this helps ensure its blood sugar–lowering benefits.

If you use insulin on a regular schedule: Exercise at the same time each day, if possible, to help maintain even, predictable blood sugar levels. Insulin should typically be used 60 to 90 minutes after your workout—check with your doctor or diabetes educator.

To prevent excessive drops in blood sugar: Eat something before or just after exercise and adjust your insulin dose on the days you work out. Talk to your doctor for specific advice.

Joint and Bone Disease

If you have arthritis, certain exercises may be painful. That's why swimming and/or aerobic exercise such as "water walking" in a warm-water pool are good options. If you don't have access to a pool, choose non–weight-bearing exercise, such as a stationary bike, to minimize stress on your joints.

With arthritis, it's especially helpful to consult your doctor or physical therapist before starting a new exercise program—so your workout can be tailored to your specific type of arthritis.

Good rule of thumb: If an exercise hurts, don't do it.

If you have bone disease, including osteoporosis or decreased bone density due to osteopenia: Weight-bearing exercise strengthens bone by exerting force against it. For this reason, walking is better than biking, for example, and swimming is usually the least likely to help.

Warning: Avoid exercises involving quick changes in direction, such as aerobic dance, which may increase fracture risk.

Lung Disease

Asthma, one of the most common lung diseases in the US, generally does not interfere with exercise unless you are performing an activity that's especially strenuous such as running, which can trigger an attack ("exercise-induced asthma").

With exercise-induced asthma, the triggers vary from person to person. For example, working out in the cold is generally to be avoided (but a face mask or scarf may warm air sufficiently). Very vigorous exercise, such as squash or mountain biking, can cause difficulties for some people with asthma, who may do better alternating brief periods of intense and slower-paced activity (as used in interval training). Know your own triggers.

Swimming is also a good choice—the high humidity helps prevent drying of the airways, which can trigger an asthma attack.

If you use an inhaler such as albuterol to treat an asthma attack: Ask your doctor about taking a dose immediately before you exercise to help prevent an attack, and always carry your inhaler with you throughout the activity.

If you have chronic obstructive pulmonary disease (COPD): Exercise doesn't improve lung function, but it does build muscle endurance and improve one's tolerance for the shortness of breath that often accompanies COPD (a condition that typically includes chronic bronchitis and/or emphysema).

Aerobic exercises that work the lower body (like walking or stationary cycling) are good, but the Schwinn Airdyne or NuStep provides a lower- and upper-body workout with the option of stopping the upper-body workout if breathing becomes more difficult.

Cancer

Exercise may help fight the nausea and muscle wasting that sometimes occur with cancer and its treatment. In fact, a recent meta-analysis of 56 studies found that aerobic exercise, including walking and cycling—both during and after treatment—reduced fatigue in cancer patients.

Interestingly, strength training was not found to reduce fatigue. But because strength training helps maintain muscle mass, some use of weights or resistance machines should be included for 15 to 20 minutes twice a week, if possible.

Because cancer patients sometimes have trouble maintaining their body weight, it's especially important for those who are exercising to increase their calorie intake to compensate for what gets burned during their workouts.

Parkinson's Disease

Regular exercise has long been known to improve symptoms and general quality of life for people with Parkinson's disease.

Now: Recent evidence shows that it may even slow progression of the disease.

Walking on a treadmill, riding a stationary bike and strength training have been shown to improve general walking speed, strength and overall fitness in

Parkinson's patients. Picking up the pace may add even more benefit—one recent study found that symptoms and brain function improved more in Parkinson's patients the faster they pedaled on a stationary bike. Tai chi and even ballroom dancing have been shown to be especially effective at improving balance in Parkinson's patients.

Keep Your Hips Forever!

Mitchell Yass, DPT, a specialist in diagnosing and resolving the cause of pain and creator of the Yass Method for treating chronic pain. He is the author of *Overpower Pain: The Strength-Training Program That Stops Pain Without Drugs or Surgery* and *The Pain Cure Rx: The Yass Method for Diagnosing and Resolving Chronic Pain.* MitchellYass.com

If you're tired of hobbling around on an aching hip, surgery to replace that failing joint might sound pretty good.

Every year, more than 330,000 Americans get this operation. For those who have severe joint damage (for example, bone-on-bone damage that prevents full range of motion), hip replacement can be an excellent choice.

Here's the rub: Many people who receive a hip replacement aren't in this category. They undergo hip replacement but don't realize that the cause of their pain could be in hip muscles, not joints.

Identify the Problem

If you complain about persistent groin pain (one of the most common symptoms of hip dysfunction), your doctor will probably order an imaging test (such as an X-ray and/or MRI scan).

What you need to know: Even though imaging tests can give doctors a great deal of information about the condition of a joint, they aren't as conclusive as you might think. For example, an X-ray can show a decrease in cartilage and less space between the thighbone and hip socket, but doctors differ in deciding at what point surgery becomes necessary. Virtually everyone who's age 50 or older will show some degree of joint damage just from normal wear and tear. A decrease in range of motion at the hip joint is key to the need for surgery.

Does a diagnosis of arthritis at the hip joint mean that you need surgery? Not necessarily. Most hip and groin pain is caused by muscle weakness or a muscle imbalance. People who correctly exercise these muscles can often eliminate—or at least greatly reduce—their discomfort. Strengthening these muscles also can help ease pain in those who have already had hip replacements...and improve balance.

The Best Workouts

The following exercises are ideal for hip or groin pain. After getting your doctor's OK, start by trying to repeat each one 10 times. Take a one-minute break, then repeat two more sets. The whole routine, which should be done two or three times a week, takes about 20 minutes.

•**Hamstring curl.** The *hamstrings* (in the back of the thigh) play a key role in the functioning of the hip joints. However, the hamstrings are weak in most people—mainly because these muscles aren't used much in normal daily movements.

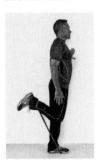

How this exercise helps: It strengthens hamstrings and helps prevent the opposing muscles (the quadriceps, in the front of the thigh) from shortening and causing muscle strain and/or spasms.

How to do it: Attach one end of a piece of elastic exercise tubing (available in sporting-goods stores and online) to your left ankle. Stand on the other end with your right foot. Leaving more slack will reduce resistance...taking up the slack will increase it.

With your feet a few inches apart and knees slightly bent, raise your left foot and curl it backward toward your buttocks as far as you comfortably can. Then return to the starting position. If you feel unsteady, put one hand (on the side opposite the leg you're working) on a wall. Switch legs and repeat.

•**Hip abduction.** This is great for hip or groin pain because the abductor muscles (on the outer thighs) tend to be much weaker than the opposing adductor muscles.

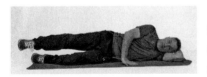

How this exercise helps: Weakness in the abductors can allow the pelvis to drop on one side, which can cause groin muscles to tighten and become painful.

How to do it: Lie on the side that's not painful (or less painful) on a mat or a carpeted floor. Your painful side will be on top. Place your arm under your head, and bend your other leg's knee for better support and balance.

Slowly raise your affected leg, keeping it in line with your torso. Keep the knee straight, and don't roll forward or backward. Raise your leg only to hip height (a few inches). Then slowly lower your leg back to the starting position. After performing a set, roll over and repeat the exercise with the other leg, only after pain has eased in the affected leg. Otherwise, focus only on strengthening the painful side.

•**Hip flexor stretch.** This exercise is vital. Most of us spend a lot of time sitting, causing these muscles to shorten and tighten.

How this exercise helps: It stretches tight hip flexors, which can stress the low back.

How to do it: Kneel on your right knee on a mat or a carpeted area. (If you need more padding, you can put a folded towel under the knee.) Place your left foot flat on the floor in front of you, with the knee bent. Rest your left hand on your left thigh and your right hand on your right hip. Keeping 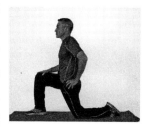 your back straight and abdominal muscles tight, lean forward so that more of your weight is on the front leg. You'll feel a stretch in your right upper thigh. Hold for 20 to 30 seconds. Switch sides.

•**Quad stretch.** Overly tight quad muscles can pull the pelvis downward—a common cause of low-back and hip pain.

How this exercise helps: Stretching the quads helps distribute weight evenly through the pelvis.

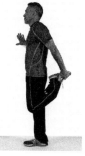

How to do it: Stand near a wall for support. Rest your right hand on the wall, then reach back with your left hand to grip your left foot/ankle. Pull your heel upward toward your buttocks— and eventually behind the hip. Keep pulling, gently, until you feel a stretch in the front of your thigh. Tighten your abdominal muscles. Hold for about 20 to 30 seconds. Repeat on the other side.

If your pain doesn't improve after a month of performing these exercises, consult your doctor.

You Need Exercise—Not a Knee Replacement

Mitchell Yass, DPT, a specialist in diagnosing and resolving the cause of pain and creator of the Yass Method for treating chronic pain. He is the author of *Overpower Pain: The Strength-Training Program That Stops Pain Without Drugs or Surgery* and *The Pain Cure Rx: The Yass Method for Diagnosing and Resolving Chronic Pain.* MitchellYass.com

D
id you know that knee-replacement surgery is virtually epidemic in this country? The number has doubled over the past decade. And among Medicare beneficiaries, the number of knee replacements has increased by more than 160%. One recent research paper reported that *4 million* Americans now have knee implants—including half a million who had to have their knee replacement redone at least once. What explains all the extra knee replacements?

It's not hard to suspect that a lot of *unnecessary operations* are being done. *So there are things you must know before letting someone cut out your knee…*

Knee-Replacement Rampage

A recent study showed that just about one-third of all knee replacements are inappropriate. The patients had relatively low levels of pain that could have been managed in other ways, and/or their knee X-rays showed little evidence of substantial arthritic changes. Many patients who were inappropriately given knee replacements were under age 55, and for them, considering that the life expectancy of the artificial joint is 15 to 20 years, another—and then perhaps another—arduous replacement operation will be needed.

Why are so many people so willingly getting an operation that is expensive, can take a year for full recovery and is certainly not without serious risks, including deadly blood clots? Most patients—and their doctors—jump to the conclusion that they need a knee replacement because of pain due to arthritis, but pain is not a reason for knee replacement or necessarily a sign of knee arthritis.

Studies that have looked at pain in relation to arthritic changes have shown that only about 15% of people with X-ray evidence of knee arthritis actually have knee pain. One study even showed that sham surgery relieved knee pain caused by osteoarthritis just as well as real surgery. Clearly the relationship between osteoarthritis and knee pain cannot be directly correlated.

The Real Cause of Knee Pain

Most people who suffer knee pain experience the pain around the kneecap. The pain is caused by an imbalance in the strength of the quadriceps muscles on the front of the thigh and the hamstring muscle on the back of it. The quadriceps naturally get a lot more use from walking and everyday activity and naturally tend to be much stronger than the hamstrings. When the hamstring muscles are weaker than the quads, the quads shorten. This increases tension on the kneecap. Instead of painlessly gliding along with the joint, the kneecap presses against the joint...painfully.

Another possible, but less likely, cause of knee pain is either a strain on the quadriceps or the band of connective tissue that runs from the hip to the outer side of the kneecap (called the *iliotibial band*). Strain on the quads will cause the kneecap to "float" outward, and strain on the iliotibial band will cause the kneecap to edge toward the left or right side of the knee joint. Either way, when the knee bends or straightens, the kneecap rubs against points in the knee joint that it shouldn't, causing pain.

The Real Solution

Joints are nothing more than "pivot points" that exist solely to allow range of motion. When a joint has undergone arthritic changes severe enough to prevent motion, then and only then is surgery warranted. To be sure, there are people whose knees have been so degraded by wear and tear that replacement is the only current option to provide them with normal use of their knee. But those people are actually rather few and far between. Rather than knee-replacement surgery, most people with knee pain need exercise to keep leg and knee muscles balanced and toned.

If you have knee pain, consider trying the exercises below to improve and balance your leg muscles and avoid the type of knee symptoms that have convinced too many people—and their doctors—that they need knee-replacement surgery. (Do check with your doctor first—but there is seldom a good medical reason not to try exercises before going to surgery.) How many reps should you do? Do each exercise 10 times, take a one-minute break, then repeat two more sets. How frequently? Two or three times a week.

•**Loosen the Quads.** Stand near a wall for support. If your left knee is the most bothersome, turn your right side to the wall and rest your right hand against it. Then, reach back with your left hand to grip your left foot or ankle. Gently pull the foot toward the buttocks until you feel a stretch in the front of your thigh. Hold for about 20 to 30 seconds. Repeat on the other side whether or not you have problems with the other knee to keep all the muscles in balance.

•**Strengthen the Hamstrings.** Practice the *straight leg dead lift*. To do this, stand with your legs hip width apart, hands at hip level either holding hand weights or grasping a pole (such a broomstick) horizontally in front of you. Bend forward from your hips, keeping your legs straight (without "locking" your knees) and letting your hands (holding weights or a pole) run down your thighs until you begin to feel a pull at the back of the thighs. Then immediately return to the start position. Do three sets of 10 repetitions.

•**Strengthen the Calves.** Strengthening the calves can help offset excessive tightening of the quads and can strengthen the hamstrings. To do this exercise, stand facing a wall, counter or sturdy chair and place both hands on it to keep your balance. Rise up onto the balls of the feet (lifting your heels)...then, gently lower your heels to the ground. Once you feel that you can keep your balance when doing this exercise, you can hold dumbbells, which will create more muscle resistance and help strengthen the calves even more.

By the third week of doing these exercises, you should notice a significant improvement. But even if you are completely rid of pain, you ought to keep up your exercise routine to keep the pain from returning. You have to keep your muscles strong your entire life to keep them functional. It's like brushing your teeth to keep decay away.

Strength Training for Beginners—No Gym Needed, No Age Limit

Cedric X. Bryant, PhD, chief science officer for the American Council on Exercise. He is author or coauthor of more than 30 books, including *Strength Training for Women.* AceFitness.org, Twitter.com/DrCedricBryant

You probably know by now that simple aerobic activity is important for cardiovascular and cognitive health, endurance, agility, weight control and all-around well-being. But (as you also probably know) maintaining muscle strength, too, is essential for good health and vitality—so here is an easy muscle-building routine suitable for seniors and newbies.

Best part: You can do it at home with just one inexpensive piece of equipment.

You have a lot to gain from this simple routine. Strength training not only builds muscles but also improves bone density, speeds up metabolism, promotes balance and even boosts brain power. This workout can also help you gain mobility.

Translation: This routine will help make everyday movements—such as getting in and out of a car, reaching overhead, bending and climbing stairs—much easier for you.

And not to worry…you won't be straining under heavy barbells. All the exercises below use just your own body weight or a simple elastic tube for resistance.

Recommended: Opt for a light-resistance tube with handles, available at sporting goods stores and online for about $10 (a good one is the durable SPRI brand, SPRI.com).

What to do: Get your doctor's OK first, as you should before beginning any new exercise routine. Perform eight to 15 reps of each of the following moves two to three times per week on nonconsecutive days—muscles need a day between workouts to repair and strengthen. Always move in a slow, controlled fashion, without jerking or using momentum. When you can easily do 15 reps of a particular exercise, advance to the "To progress" variation.

No-Equipment-Needed Exercises…

- **Wall Squat—for legs and buttocks.**

Start: Stand with head and back against a wall, arms at sides, legs straight, feet hip-width apart and about 18 inches from wall.

Move: Keeping head and torso upright and your back firmly pressed against the wall, bend knees and slide down the wall about four to eight inches. Knees should be aligned above ankles—do not allow knees to extend past toes. Hold for several seconds. Then, using thigh and buttock muscles, straighten legs and slide back up wall to the start position. Repeat.

To progress: Bend knees more, ideally to a 90° angle so thighs are parallel to floor, as if sitting in a chair. http://bit.ly/19uRM9.

- **Wall Pushup—for chest, shoulders and triceps.**

Start: Stand facing a wall, feet hip-width apart and about 18 inches from wall. Place hands on wall at shoulder height, slightly wider than shoulder-width apart.

Move: Tighten abdominal muscles to brace your midsection, keeping spine and legs straight throughout. Slowly bend elbows, bringing face as close to wall as you can. Hold for one second, then straighten arms and return to the start position. Repeat.

To progress: Start with feet farther from wall…and bring face closer to wall during pushup. http://bit.ly/11hnyM.

• **Supine Reverse March—for abdominals, lower back and hips.**

Start: Lie face up, knees bent, feet flat on floor, arms out to sides in a T position, palms up, abs contracted.

Move: Slowly lift left foot off floor, keeping leg bent…bring knee up and somewhat closer to torso…when left thigh is vertical to floor, stop moving and hold for five to 10 seconds. Then slowly lower leg and return foot to floor. Repeat. Switch legs.

To progress: As knee moves upward, raise both arms toward ceiling… lower arms as leg lowers. AceFitness.org/exercise-library-details/0/238/.

Moves with Tubes…

• **Seated Row—for back, abs and biceps.**

Start: Sit on floor, torso upright, legs out in front of you, knees slightly bent, feet together. Place center of elastic resistance tube across soles of feet and hold tube handles in hands, arms extended in front of you, elbows straight.

Move: Bending elbows, slowly pull handles of tube toward chest (do not lean backward, arch back, shrug shoulders or bend wrists). Hold for several seconds, then slowly straighten arms and return to the start position. Repeat.

To progress: To increase resistance, rather than placing center of tube across soles of feet, anchor it firmly around an immovable object one to three feet in front of you.

• **Lateral Raise—for shoulders.**

Start: Stand with feet hip-width apart, anchoring center of elastic resistance tube under both feet. Hold tube handles in hands, arms down at sides.

Move: Keeping elbows very slightly bent and wrists straight, slowly lift arms out to sides so palms face floor and hands reach shoulder height (or as high as you can get them). Lower arms to the start position. Repeat.

To progress: To increase resistance, widen your stance on the tubing. http://bit.ly/PdpD Lw.

Keep Your Hands Young and Strong

Anjum Lone, OTR/L, CHT, an occupational and certified hand therapist and chief of the department of occupational therapy at Phelps Memorial Hospital Center in Sleepy Hollow, New York.

I f you have been diagnosed with arthritis, it's wise to protect your hands right away.

Both osteoarthritis (known as "wear-and-tear" arthritis) and rheumatoid arthritis (an autoimmune disease) can damage cartilage and sometimes the bones themselves.

Daily hand exercises can improve joint lubrication…increase your range of motion and hand strength…and maintain or restore function. These exercises also are helpful for people who have a hand injury or who heavily use their hands.

Save Your Hands with Exercise

Most hand and wrist exercises can be done at home without equipment. But don't exercise during flare-ups, particularly if you have rheumatoid arthritis. Patients who ignore the pain and overuse their hands and wrists are more likely to suffer long-term damage, including joint deformity.

Important: Warm the joints before doing these exercises—this helps prevent micro-tears that can occur when stretching cold tissue. Simply run warm water over your hands in the sink for a few minutes right before the exercises. Or you can warm them with a heating pad.

Before doing the hand exercises here, it also helps to use the fingers of the other hand to rub and knead the area you'll be exercising. This self-massage improves circulation to the area and reduces swelling.

If you have osteoarthritis or rheumatoid arthritis, do the following exercises five times on each hand—and work up to 10 times, if possible. The entire sequence should take no more than five minutes. Perform the sequence two to three times a day.*

1. Tendon glides.

Purpose: Keeps the tendons functioning well to help move all the finger joints through their full range of motion.

What to do: Rest your elbow on a table with your forearm and hand raised (fingertips pointed to the ceiling). Bend the fingers at the middle joint (form a hook with your fingers), and hold this position for a moment. Then bend the fingers into a fist, hiding your nails. Don't clench—just fold your fingers gently while keeping the wrist in a "neutral" position. Now make a modified fist with your nails 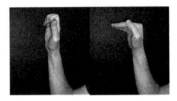 showing. Next, raise your fingers so that they are bent at a 90-degree angle and your thumb is resting against your index finger (your hand will look similar to a bird's beak). Hold each position for three seconds.

2. Thumb active range of motion.

Purpose: Improves your ability to move your thumb in all directions. Do the movements gently so that you don't feel any pain.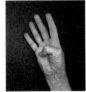

What to do: Rest your elbow on a table with your forearm and hand in the air. Touch the tip of the thumb to the tip of each finger (or get as close as you can). Then, flex the tip of your thumb toward the palm. Hold each of these positions for three seconds.

3. Web-space massage.

Purpose: Using one hand to massage the other hand strengthens muscles in the "active" hand while increasing circulation in the "passive" hand.

What to do: Clasp your left hand with your right hand as if you are shaking hands. With firm but gentle pressure, use the length of your left thumb to massage the web (space between the thumb and the index finger) next to your right thumb. Then, reverse the position and massage the web next to your left thumb. Massage each web for 30 seconds.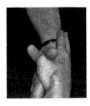

*For more exercises, see an occupational therapist. To find one, consult the American Occupational Therapy Association, AOTA.org.

4. Wrist active range of motion.

Purpose: To maintain proper positioning of the wrist, which helps keep the fingers in correct alignment.

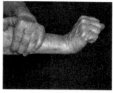

What to do: Rest your right forearm on a table with your wrist hanging off the edge and your palm pointing downward—you'll only be moving your wrist. Then place your left hand on top of your right forearm to keep it stable. With the fingers on your right hand held together gently, raise the wrist as high as it will comfortably go. Hold for three seconds.

Next, make a fist and raise it so the knuckles point upward. Now, lower the fist toward the floor. Hold each position for three seconds.

5. Digit extension.

Purpose: Strengthens the muscles that pull the fingers straight—the movement prevents chronic contractions that can lead to joint deformity.

What to do: Warm up by placing the palms and fingers of both hands together and pressing the hands gently for five seconds. Then place your palms flat on a table. One at a time, raise each finger. Then lift all the fingers on one hand simultaneously while keeping your palm flat on the table. Hold each movement for five seconds.

6. Wrist flexion/extension.

Purpose: Stretches and promotes muscle length in the forearm. Forearm muscles move the wrist and fingers. Flexion (bending your wrist so that your palm approaches the forearm) and extension (bending your wrist in the opposite direction) help maintain wrist strength and range of motion.

What to do: Hold your right hand in the air, palm down. Bend the wrist upward so that the tips of your fingers are pointed toward the ceiling. Place your left hand against the fingers (on the palm side) and gently push so that the back of your right hand moves toward the top of your right forearm. Hold for 15 seconds. Switch hands and repeat.

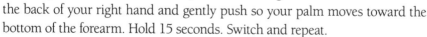

Now, bend your right wrist downward so that the fingers are pointed at the floor. Place your left hand against the back of your right hand and gently push so your palm moves toward the bottom of the forearm. Hold 15 seconds. Switch and repeat.

7. Finger-walking exercises.

Purpose: Strengthens fingers in the opposite direction of a deformity. This exercise is particularly helpful for rheumatoid arthritis patients.

What to do: Put one hand on a flat surface. Lift the index finger up and move it toward the thumb, then place the finger down. Next, lift the middle finger and move it toward the index finger. Lift the ring finger and move it toward the middle finger. Finally, lift the little finger and move it toward the ring finger. Repeat on your other hand.

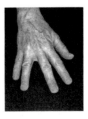

CHAPTER 4

Grow Younger: Look Good and Feel Good

12 Things That Make You Look Older

Kim Johnson Gross, cocreator of the *Chic Simple* book series and author of *What to Wear for the Rest of Your Life*. KimJohnsonGross.com

As you get older, wardrobe and style choices that worked when you were younger may no longer be serving you well. This goes for both men and women. Without knowing it, you may be looking older than you are. This could cause others to treat you as older and potentially hold you back from employment opportunities and advancements. This also can make you feel like you are not up to your game or comfortable in your skin. When you are not style confident, you are less body confident, which makes you feel less life confident.

Helpful: Seek out style mentors—people who look elegant and modern without chasing youth-oriented trends. Observe them carefully, and adapt elements of their style to your own. TV newscasters make good style mentors because they are required to look contemporary while also projecting dignity and authority.

Give yourself a good, hard look, and ask yourself whether you are looking older than your actual age with any of these common signals…

1. Sneakers for everyday wear. Your feet should be comfortable, but sneakers outside the gym just look sloppy and careless. Young people get away with it—but there are more stylish options when you're older. These include loafers or driving moccasins for men and low-heeled pumps with cushioned soles for women. Wedge-soled shoes are a comfortable alternative to high heels.

2. Baggy pants. Although young men may look trendy in high-waisted, loose-fitting jeans, this style screams old on anyone else. For women, the rear end tends to flatten with age, causing pants to fit loosely in the rear. And front-pleated pants for women generally are unflattering and unstylish.

Better: Spend the time to find pants that fit well—or figure a tailor into your wardrobe budget. Baggy is dowdy, but overly tight makes you look heavier. Well-fitting clothes make you look slimmer and younger.

3. Boring colors. Skin tone gets duller with age, so the colors you wear should bring light to your face. If you are a woman who has worn black for years, it may be too harsh for you now. Brown makes men fade into the woodwork.

Better: Stand in front of a mirror, and experiment with colors that you never thought you could wear—you may be surprised at what flatters you. Avoid neon brights, which make older skin look sallow, but be open to the rest of the color spectrum. Try contemporary patterns and prints. For neutrals, gray and navy are softer alternatives to black for women, and any shade of blue is a good bet for men.

4. Boring glasses and jewelry. Men and women should have some fun with glasses. It's a great way to update your look and make it more modern. Tell your optician what you're looking for, or bring a stylish friend with you.

As for jewelry for women, wearing a large piece of fab faux jewelry (earrings, necklace, ring) or multiple bracelets adds great style and youth to your look.

5. Turtlenecks. You may think a turtleneck hides a sagging neck and chin, but it is more likely to draw attention to jowls.

Better: A cowl neckline for women, or a loosely draped scarf. A scarf is the single best item to help a woman look thinner, taller, prettier and more chic. You can find several scarf instructional videos online. We like Nordstrom's "How to Tie a Scarf" (search YouTube). For a man, an oblong scarf, looped, is a stylish European look that adds a welcome shot of color.

6. Stiff or one-tone hair. An overly styled helmet of hair looks old-fashioned. Hair that's a solid block of color looks unnatural and harsh.

Better: Whether hair is short or shoulder-length, women need layers around the face for softness. As for color, opt for subtle highlights in front and a slightly darker tone toward the back.

Keep in mind that gray hair can be beautiful, modern and sexy. You need a plan to go gray, though, which means a flattering cut and using hair products that enhance the gray. Ask your stylist for recommendations. Also, if your hair is a dull gray, consider getting silver highlights around your face to bring light and "energy" to your hair.

Men who dye their hair should allow a bit of gray at the temples—it looks more natural than monochrome hair. But avoid a comb-over or a toupee. A man who attempts to hide a receding hairline isn't fooling anyone—he just looks insecure.

Better: Treat your thinning hair as a badge of honor. Either keep it neatly trimmed or shave your head.

7. Missing (or bushy) eyebrows. Women's eyebrows tend to disappear with age. Men's are more likely to grow wild.

Better: Women should use eyebrow pencil, powder or both to fill in fading brows. Visit a high-end cosmetics counter, and ask the stylist to show you how. You may need to try several products to find out what works best. Men, make sure that your barber or hair stylist trims your eyebrows regularly.

Also: Women tend not to notice increased facial hair (especially stray hairs) on the chin and upper lip—a result of hormonal change. Pluck!

8. Deeply tanned skin. Baby boomers grew up actively developing suntans using baby oil and sun reflectors. Now pale is the norm. A dark tan not only dates you, it increases your risk for skin cancer and worsens wrinkling.

Better: Wear a hat and sunscreen to shield your skin from sun damage.

9. Less-than-white teeth. Yellowing teeth add decades to your appearance. Everyone's teeth get yellower with age, but with so many teeth-whitening products available, there is no excuse to live with off-color teeth.

Better: Ask your dentist which whitening technique he/she recommends based on the condition of your teeth—over-the-counter whitening strips, bleaching in the dentist's office or a custom bleaching kit you can use at home.

10. Women: Nude or beige hose. Nude stockings on women look hopelessly out-of-date. Bare legs are the norm now for young women, but they are not a good option for older women who have dark veins.

Better: In winter, wear dark stockings or opaque tights. In summer, use spray-on tanner for a light tan...or wear nude fishnet stockings or slacks or capris.

11. Poor-fitting bra. Get a bra that fits. Most women don't know that bra size changes as your body does. Giving your breasts a lift will make you look younger and trimmer.

12. Excess makeup. Thick foundation, heavy eyeliner, bright blusher and red lipstick all add years to your face.

Better: Use a moisturizing (not matte) foundation, and dab it only where needed to even out skin tone. To add color to cheeks, use a small amount of tinted moisturizer, bronzer or cream blush. Use liquid eyeliner in soft shades such as deep blue or brown, and blend it well. For lips, choose soft pinks and mauves, depending on your skin tone.

Bottom line: The idea is to have fun putting yourself together. That inner spark and personal style will show that you are getting better with age.

Skin Care from the Inside Out

Joy Bauer, MS, RD, CDN, a nutritionist/dietitian in private practice in New York City. She is author of several books, including *Joy Bauer's Food Cures: Treat Common Health Concerns, Look Younger & Live Longer.* JoyBauer.com

To take care of their skin, most people reach for sunscreen, lotions and creams to protect, smooth and moisturize. These products can help, but beautiful, healthy skin starts with what goes into your body, not what you rub on it. Research shows that good nutrition may reduce the effects of sun damage…minimize redness and wrinkling…and even protect against some skin cancers.

First Step: Hydrate

The single most important nutritional factor for keeping skin healthy is water. Staying hydrated keeps cells plump, making skin look firmer and clearer. When cells are dehydrated, they shrivel and can make your skin look wrinkled. Think of it this way—when you dehydrate a juicy grape, you get a raisin. In addition, water transports nutrients into skin cells and helps flush toxins out of the body.

To stay hydrated, drink whenever you feel thirsty.

Helpful sign: If your urine is pale yellow, you are adequately hydrated— but if it is bright or dark yellow, you may need to boost your fluid intake.

Good news: Drinking unsweetened tea helps keep you hydrated, plus you get the benefit of antioxidant nutrients called polyphenols, which may help prevent sun-related skin cancers. Green, white, black and oolong teas provide more polyphenols than herbal teas. It is your choice whether to drink caffeinated or decaffeinated tea. Although caffeine is a mild diuretic (increasing the amount of urine that is passed from the body), the relatively small amount in tea doesn't affect its ability to keep skin hydrated and healthy.

Avoid: Teas sweetened with a lot of sugar—excess sugar can make skin dull and wrinkled.

For extra hydration: Eat "juicy foods" that are at least 75% water by weight—fruits such as apples, berries, cherries, grapes, grapefruit, mangoes, melons, oranges, peaches, plums…and vegetables such as asparagus, beets, carrots, celery, cucumbers and tomatoes.

Skin-Healthy Foods

Everything we eat is reflected in the health of our skin—for better or for worse. *Among the best nutrients for the skin…*

•**Beta-carotene,** a powerful antioxidant that, once ingested, is converted to vitamin A, a nutrient necessary for skin tissue growth and repair.

Skin-smart: Have at least one serving per day of beta-carotene–rich foods— for instance, orange carrots, sweet potatoes and tomatoes…green arugula, asparagus and spinach…and fruits such as cherries, grapefruit, mangoes and watermelon.

•**Omega-3 fatty acids,** healthful fats that are important building blocks of the membranes that make up cell walls, allowing water and nutrients to enter and keeping out waste and toxins.

Skin-smart: Eat at least three servings of omega-3–rich foods each week— such as wild salmon (farm-raised salmon may have higher levels of potentially dangerous contaminants)…mackerel (not king mackerel, which has too much mercury)…anchovies, herring and sardines. Good fats also are found in smaller amounts in flaxseed, soybeans and walnuts. If you don't eat enough of these omega-3 foods, consider taking daily supplements of fish oil providing 1,000 mg of combined eicosapentaenoic acid (EPA) and docosahexaenoic acid (DHA), the most biologically active and beneficial components. Look for brands that have been tested for purity, such as Ultimate Omega by Nordic Naturals (NordicNaturals.com).

•**Selenium,** a mineral with antioxidant activity thought to help skin elasticity (which means you'll look younger longer) and prevent sun-related skin damage and cancers.

Skin-smart: Eat at least one serving a day of a selenium-rich food—canned light tuna (which has less mercury than canned albacore or white tuna), crab, tilapia…whole-wheat breads and pasta…lean beef…chicken and turkey (breast meat is lowest in fat).

Caution: Taking selenium in supplement form may increase the risk for squamous cell skin cancer in people with a personal or family history of the disease. Selenium in food is safe and healthful.

•**Vitamin C,** an antioxidant that helps build collagen and elastin (proteins that comprise the skin's underlying structure)…and also protects against free radicals (molecules in the body that damage cells) when the skin is exposed to sunlight.

Skin-smart: Eat at least one serving a day of any of these vitamin C-rich foods—cantaloupe, citrus fruits, kiwifruit, papaya, pineapple, strawberries, watermelon…and bell peppers, broccoli, brussels sprouts, cabbage, cauliflower, kale and kidney beans.

•**Zinc,** a mineral that helps maintain collagen. People with zinc deficiencies often develop skin redness and lesions.

Skin-smart: Eat at least one serving of a zinc-rich food daily—chicken or turkey breast, crab, lean beef, pork tenderloin (lower in fat than other cuts)…peanuts and peanut butter…fat-free dairy products (cheese, milk and yogurt).

Wise for everyone: A daily multivitamin that contains 100% of the daily value for vitamins A, C, E and zinc and no more than 70 mcg of selenium.

How You Can Stand Taller As You Age

Joel Harper, personal trainer, has designed custom workouts for celebrities and Olympic medalists, and is the creator of the PBS DVD, *Firming Up After 50*. He is based in New York City. JoelHarperFitness.com

Here's a simple antiaging trick that will make you look and feel much younger (and costs nothing at all!)—stand straight and tall. Unfortunately, as you age and your muscles get weaker, this becomes more challenging. Here's a routine that builds strength all over your body, takes just 10 minutes a day and delivers a noticeable improvement in posture in just a few weeks.

Not sure whether you need it? Here's a test…With your back against the wall, slide down to sit in an imaginary chair, legs bent, heels directly underneath your knees and thighs parallel to the floor. (If this makes you feel uncomfortable or unsteady, don't try to slide down this far—you've already learned that you could benefit from this routine!) People with reasonably good posture can easily rest the back of their heads and shoulders against the wall in this "chair" position for one full minute...so if you can't, you've got work to do.

Do each of these three pairs in a row every other day for two weeks. Of course, if there's any chance that trying new exercises might not be safe for you, check these with your doctor first.

Posture Pairing #1

"Field goals" strengthen your shoulders. With your back against a wall, stand with feet together and raise your arms at your sides to make a "T." Then bend your elbows and raise your forearms, forming a 90-degree angle with your palms facing forward and fingers spread. Now lower your hands to make your forearms horizontal—and repeat this last motion, both sides at the same time, 25 times. Resist moving your elbows. Keep your shoulders relaxed, not shrugged. You can add a balance component to this exercise by slightly lifting your heels as you do the arm movements and/or pump it up by adding three-pound hand weights.

"Chicken wing" stretches your shoulders and upper back. Standing up straight with your stomach pulled in, put your left hand on your left hip, fingers behind you. Now reach your right hand in front of your body to grasp your left elbow and gently pull it toward your stomach. That'll stretch the left side of your arm, upper back and shoulders. Hold where you feel the stretch and take five deep breaths...then switch sides and repeat. If one side is tighter than the other, repeat on that side, with the goal of eventually making both sides equal.

Posture Pairing #2

"Rickety table" strengthens the back, arms and glutes. Get down on all fours on a padded surface, with your fingers spread apart, making sure your hands are in line with your shoulders and your knees with your hips. Keep your back flat and parallel to the floor. With your left arm slightly bent (so you work the muscle, not the joint), reach your right arm straight forward and your left foot straight back, stretching them as far away from each other as possible, aiming to keep your right hand one inch higher than your head. Hold for 25 seconds. Work up to that amount of time if you can't do it at first. Or, if this move feels too easy, then simultaneously lower your right hand and left foot (big toe) to tap them on the floor and then raise them back to horizontal position. Repeat this 25 times, then switch sides. An even more advanced version is to tap your elbow to the opposite knee (instead of tapping your hand and foot on the ground) and then return to parallel position after each tap.

"Elbow circling" releases tension and stretches muscles in your shoulders and neck. You can do this either sitting or standing. Put your right fingertips on top of your right shoulder and your left fingertips on top of your left shoulder and then touch your elbows together in front of you. Keeping your fingers where they are and looking straight ahead, make large circles toward the outside of your body with each elbow simultaneously. Inhale on one circle on a count of five and exhale on the next count of five. Do six circles in that direction, and then do six in the opposite direction. This is great to do if you sit at a desk all day.

Posture Pairing #3

"Side-lying kick" strengthens the oblique (side) abdominal and leg muscles. Lie on the ground on your left side, stretching your left arm above your head so that your left ear rests on your arm. Keeping your stomach taut and resisting rocking, bend your left knee to a 45-degree angle with your heel in line with your spine. Lift your right (straight) leg three-feet directly above your left foot... then tap your right knee lightly on the ground in front of your waist. Then lift your leg back up, straighten it and kick three feet in the air above your left foot (or as high as you can). Do this sequence 25 times and then switch sides.

"Airplane stretch" stretches the hips and legs. While seated on a straight-backed chair or stool, put the right side of your right foot onto your left knee. Rest your right elbow on top of your right knee and your right hand on your right ankle. While keeping your back straight, gently lean forward. Look straight ahead. You can increase the stretch by using your left hand to gently turn the sole of your right foot to face up. Hold for 30 seconds, taking deep breaths. Switch sides and repeat. If you find that one side of your body is tighter than the other, then you should repeat on that particular side in order to create balance.

A Final Tip

An easy way to keep your posture picture-perfect is to always try to keep your gaze straight ahead. It's almost impossible to have bad posture if you keep your eyes at eye level. It's a simple trick to keep in mind as you go about your busy day, looking younger and feeling great!

CHAPTER 5

Age Well in Your Home

High-Tech Ways to Age at Home

Majd Alwan, PhD, senior vice president of technology and executive director of the LeadingAge Center for Aging Services Technologies, a nonprofit for aging advocacy in Washington, DC. LeadingAge.org/CAST

Where do you plan to live during your retirement years—including your latest years? If you're like most people, you want to stay right at home.

But that doesn't work for everyone. People with chronic illnesses and/or physical disabilities may end up moving into assisted-living facilities or nursing homes—and often sooner than they had hoped.

Now: High-tech devices can help you stay in your home much longer than before (even if you live alone) while also giving loved ones the assurance that you are safe.

To stay at home as long as possible, people have traditionally installed ramps, grab bars, brighter lighting and other such products to accommodate their changing needs. But that doesn't scratch the surface of what's available today.

Impressive high-tech devices to help you stay at home as you age…

"Checkups" at Home

There's now an easy way to quickly alert your doctor of important changes in your health that may be occurring between office visits.

What's new: Remote patient monitoring. You can use an at-home glucose monitor, weight scale, pulse oximeter (to measure oxygen in the blood) and other devices that store readings, which you can then easily share with your doctor—on a daily, weekly or monthly basis, depending on your condition and how well you're responding to treatments.

Example: A wireless glucose monitor, such as the iHealth Align ($16.95, for smartphone, $29.99, for separate monitor), available at iHealthLabs.com. It works with a smartphone to take glucose readings and automatically log/track measurements over time and send them to the doctor.

Fall Monitors Go High-Tech

We're all familiar with the older fall-monitor systems that require users to press a button on a pendant to initiate communication with a call center. Staffers then contact you (via an intercom-like device) to ask if you need help.

What's new: Devices that don't require the push of a button, so fall victims who are immobilized or unconscious also can be helped.

New-generation fall monitors are equipped with accelerometers that can tell when you've fallen. The units, worn around the neck, on the wrist or clipped to a belt, contact a call center or a designated caregiver. If you don't answer a follow-up call, emergency responders will be sent to your address.

Why the new technology is important: Fall victims who receive help within one hour of a fall are six times more likely to survive than those who wait longer.

Examples: Philips Lifeline HomeSafe with AutoAlert (automatic fall detection with push-button backup, 24-hour call center/emergency response) starts at $29.95/month. GoSafe is a wireless version that starts at $44.95/month, plus a onetime GoSafe mobile button purchase of $99.95. Both are available at Life Line.Philips.com.

Traditional-style fall monitor: Walgreens Ready Response Vi Alert System (390-foot range, 24-hour call center/emergency response) requires the fall victim to push a button. Available at WalgreensReadyResponse.com for $29.99/month (866-310-9061).

Activity Monitors

By tracking activity—and noting changes in routines—an off-site loved one or caregiver can tell when you've become more or less active or when you're spending more time in certain parts of the house. A sudden increase in bathroom visits, for example, could indicate a urinary tract infection that hasn't yet been diagnosed.

What's new: Sensors that track daily activity—for example, how often refrigerator doors are opened, when the stove is turned on and how often the bathroom is used.

Examples: GrandCare Activity Monitoring Package. A caregiver can log in to the system to view activity reports and/or set up "alert parameters" that will trigger an alert if there is no registered movement at scheduled times. A personalized package is available at GrandCare.com, starting at $299.99, plus a monthly fee based on system developed.

Another option is Wellness Solutions by Alarm.com. Sensors are installed throughout the home to detect activity and any abnormal changes in routine. Alerts are sent via a smartphone app. Consumers can buy the sensors from local dealers in a variety of packages, starting at $99. Visit Alarm.com (click "Wellness" under "Products & Services") to locate a dealer near you.

How's Your Walking

A change in walking speed could indicate that someone has balance problems, muscle weakness or other issues that can interfere with daily living.

What's new: Wearable devices (available from your doctor or physical therapist) that monitor gait, balance and walking speed. The devices store information that can be electronically transmitted to a doctor or physical therapist.

If walking speed has declined, it could mean that an underlying health problem—such as congestive heart failure—isn't well controlled by medication…or that you need physical therapy to increase muscle strength and stamina. Detecting such changes in gait in high-risk patients can allow treatment adjustments that help prevent falls and improve mobility—critical for staying (and thriving) at home.

Examples: StepWatch from Modus Health straps onto your ankle and has 27 different metrics to measure gait and speed. Available at ModusHealth. com. LEGSys from Biosensics includes portable, wireless sensors that analyze gait and generate easy-to-read reports. It's easy to put on with a Velcro strap. Available at Biosensics.com/products/LEGSys.

30 Handy Aids for Achy Hands

Jim Miller, an advocate for older Americans, writes "Savvy Senior," a weekly information column syndicated in more than 400 newspapers nationwide. Based in Norman,
Oklahoma, he also offers a free senior news service at SavvySenior.org.

People typically don't think about how much they use their hands until
their hands get stiff and painful.

Arthritis, carpal tunnel syndrome and other conditions can make
performing everyday tasks such as turning a doorknob, fastening a button,
brushing your teeth, preparing a meal or using a computer mouse difficult and
painful. There are various assistive devices and other products to help ease the
burden of having achy hands. *Here are some of the best ones...*

Kitchen Aids

•**Dexter DuoGlide Knives** have soft, textured handles and curved blades
that let you chop foods using a rocking motion with less hand strain. Available in six models—paring knife, utility knife, bread slicer, all-purpose knife,
cook's knife and chef's knife. From $22.50 to $64.85.* Dexter1818.com (800-
343-6042).

•**Anolon 14-Inch French Skillet** ($59.99) and **Circulon 6-Quart Covered
Chef Pan** ($79.99) both have a large, ergonomically designed handle and a sec-
ond helper handle on each pan that makes them easier to lift and move around
when cooking, cleaning or serving. PotsAndPans.com

•**West Bend Electric Can Opener** is a hands-free can opener that starts
and stops automatically once you lock the can in place. A built-in magnet keeps
the lid from falling in the food once open. $45.99. WestBend.com

•**Zim Jar Opener** has a V-shaped grip that holds the lid still as you use both
hands to twist open a jar or bottle. Available in wall-mounted ($17.99) and
under-counter-mounted ($16.99) versions, these openers require installation.
Amazon.com

Alternative: **Hamilton Beach Open Ease Automatic Jar Opener** is a
small, battery-operated device that opens twist-lids from one to four inches
in diameter at the push of a button. $34.95. Amazon.com

*Prices and product models subject to change.

•**Good Grips Eating Utensils** (fork, small spoon, teaspoon, tablespoon, soupspoon and rocker knife) are stainless steel with large, soft 1⅜-inch, non-slip grips that are easy to grasp. The fork and spoons also have a special twist built into the metal shaft that allows them to be bent to any angle for either left- or right-handed use, which helps people with limited hand-to-mouth reach. $10.95 per utensil. NCmedical.com

•**OXO Good Grips** makes easy-to-grip cooking and baking utensils with large, soft handles. They range from spatulas and whisks to pizza wheels and ice cream scoops. Large-handled utensils spread your fingers so that they don't close completely around the tool, which reduces hand stress and makes the utensils more comfortable to grasp. Typically from $5 to $13 per item. OXO.com

Household Helpers

•**Lever faucet handles.** If you have twist-handle kitchen or bathroom faucets, check the brand and then see if lever-styled replacement handles are available through the manufacturer's website or through a home-improvement store. Lever handles provide greater leverage for easier turning.

Example: Danco Decorative Lever Handle, $14.98 each at The Home Depot. If lever-style replacement handles are not available, replace your faucets with lever-handle faucets.

The following items can be found at Amazon.com…

•**Door Knob Grippers** fit over standard doorknobs, converting them into easy-to-turn door levers. $10.69 for a package of two.

•**Key turners** attach to a key. Each turner has two finger holes in the handle to improve grip and leverage. $7.95.

•**Big lamp switch** is a large, three-spoked knob adapter that provides better leverage for turning a lamp switch. $10.35.

Personal Care

•**Simplehuman triple wall-mount pump** holds liquid soap, shampoo and conditioner and has a T-bar lever at the base of each container that you pull for one-handed dispensing. $70. Simplehuman.com

•**Simplehuman sensor pump** is a touch-free liquid-hand-soap dispenser that sits by the kitchen or bathroom sink. Place your hand under the spout to dispense the soap automatically. $40. Simplehuman.com

•**Touch N Brush: The Hands-Free Toothpaste Dispenser** can hold any size tube of toothpaste and attaches to the bathroom mirror or the wall with suction cups. Just touch the pump arm with your toothbrush head to get a strip of toothpaste without squeezing the tube. $27.95. Amazon.com

•**Oral-B and Sonicare** offer a variety of electric toothbrushes with handles that are easier to hold and are wider than standard manual brushes. Prices for the Oral-B toothbrushes run between $39.99 and $169.99 (OralB.com). Sonicare toothbrushes cost between $39.95 and $189.95 (USA.Philips.com).

Cheaper alternative: Foam tubing can be cut down to size and fit onto your toothbrush handle to create a large, soft handgrip. This also can be used on eating utensils, pens and pencils. Available in ¼-inch, ⅜-inch and 1⅛-inch widths, this tubing is slip-resistant and does not absorb water. $14.35. Maddak.com

•**Philips Sonicare AirFloss** cleans between your teeth by shooting microbursts of air and water droplets, eliminating the need for string floss. $49.99. USA.Philips.com (800-682-7664).

Easier Dressing

•**Dressing aid with shoe horn** on one end helps guide your heel into shoes, boots and slippers, saving you from bending and reaching. Opposite end features dressing hooks that help you pull on socks, shoes, pants and tops without straining. $8.99. EasyComforts.com

•**Zipper pulls** are three-inch-long polypropylene pulls that attach to zipper tabs, making them easier to grasp. $4.99 for a set of 12 in assorted colors. EasyComforts.com

•**Lock Laces** are elastic shoelaces that convert lace-ups into slip-ons. To ensure a good fit, they include a spring-activated locking device that can tighten and loosen the shoelaces. Available in a variety of colors for $7.99 or $9.99 per pair. LockLaces.com

Easier Driving

These are available at Amazon.com…

•**Car key turner** (around $6) is a curved, five-inch-long plastic handle that attaches to the key to provide leverage.

•**Gas cap removal tool** ($15) works like a wrench and fits most gas caps.

•**Steering wheel cover** ($10 to $22) fits over the steering wheel to make the wheel larger in size and easier to grip. There are numerous options, including heated versions.

Reading, Writing and Computing

For book readers, electronic e-readers are ideal because they're lightweight and easier to hold than regular books and don't require traditional page turning. But if you like paper publications, there are bookholders such as **Levo Book Holder Floor Stand** ($169) and **Corner Table Clamp Book Holder** ($99) that hold hardcovers, paperbacks, magazines and cookbooks in any position. Levo also offers holders for e-readers and tablet computers that cost between $99.99 and $229.99. Levostore. com

•**The Pencil Grip** is a small rubber grip that fits on pencils and pens to make holding easier and reduce hand fatigue. $1.79. ThePencilGrip.com

•**Pen Again** is a Y-shaped pen that cradles your index finger to relieve hand stress when writing. $4.99. PenAgain.net

•**3M Ergonomic Mouse** has a vertical-grip handle design that keeps your arm in a more neutral position to reduce wrist and hand stress when using a computer. $58.57. Amazon.com

•**Contour RollerMouse** sits directly in front of the computer keyboard, giving you the ability to control the cursor with your fingertips, eliminating the reaching and gripping of a traditional mouse. $199.95 to $265. Contour Design.com

---

Are You Afraid of Falling?

Those who are afraid of falling are also more likely to avoid everyday activities such as walking outside, shopping for groceries or taking a bath…and are far more likely to end up in a nursing home.

Here's a quick rule of thumb: If you've had two or fewer minor falls in the past year…if you don't walk more slowly than other people your age…and if you can stand up from a chair without using your arms, you probably don't need to limit your activities dramatically due to concern about falling. However, if you are more afraid of falling than you need to be, it's important to take steps to reduce your fear. (See chapter 6, "Secrets to Staying Steady on Your Feet" for ways to protect from falling.)

Julie Wetherell, PhD, a board-certified geropsychologist at the VA San Diego Healthcare System and professor of psychiatry at the University of California, San Diego.

Low-Cost Ways to Make Your Home Easier and Safer to Live In

Tom Kraeutler, a former professional home inspector and contractor in New York City. He is host of *The Money Pit*, a nationally syndicated radio show on home improvement broadcast to more than three million listeners. MoneyPit.com

Ella Chadwell, a home-safety consultant, Brentwood, Tennessee, and president of Life@Home, a web-based company that provides information on home-accident prevention and markets products for home safety.

Wendy A. Jordan, a Certified Aging-in-Place Specialist (CAPS), designated by the National Association of Home Builders.

Remodeling a house to make it safer and more user-friendly can run tens of thousands of dollars. *But here are ways* to improve and update your home without spending much…*

Throughout the Home

•**Replace round doorknobs,** which are difficult to grasp and turn, with lever-style handles that you push down to open. Most of the time, the lever handles can be attached to the existing latch mechanism already on the door. You can do the job yourself with just a screwdriver. Also, consider replacing cabinet door and drawer knobs with easy-to-grasp C- or D-shaped handles.

Cost: About $30/lever and $10/handle. Available at home-improvement centers.

•**Install better lighting.** Vision inevitably deteriorates with age. Adequate lighting throughout the house helps prevent falls and run-ins with walls, corners and doors. Central ceiling fixtures, wall sconces with translucent shades and skylights are all good choices. Motion-activated lighting is helpful during middle-of-the-night trips to the bathroom. Task lighting in the bathroom, kitchen and reading nooks should be directed from the side, versus overhead, to avoid glare.

Cost: Average $95 to $1,500, depending on scope of work done.

*Most of these items are widely available at home-improvement and plumbing-supply stores. For proper installation, consult an occupational therapist or Certified Aging-in-Place Specialist (CAPS)—architects, designers, contractors and health-care consultants with special training in modifying homes for older individuals. To find a CAPS in your area, go to NAHB.org/capsdirectory.

●**Switch to rocker light switches.** They are on/off switches that rock back and forth when pressed. They are larger and easier to operate, and many people find them more attractive than the standard, small flip switches used in most homes. Rocker switches let you turn on a light with your elbow or fist if you're entering a room when your hands are full, and they're easier to find in the dark.

Cost: About $5 per light switch. Available at home-improvement centers.

●**Raise the position of some electrical outlets.** Wall outlets that are close to the floor can be hard to reach and inconvenient for plugging in appliances that you use intermittently, such as vacuums, heating pads and chargers for phones and laptops. Use those low outlets for lamps and other devices that you rarely unplug. Hire an electrician to raise other outlets at least 27 inches off the floor. They'll still be inconspicuous but much more accessible.

Cost: Typically $250 and up to move about half a dozen outlets.

●**Use remote controls for more than TVs.** They can operate window coverings, such as drapes and blinds, so you avoid stretching and straining, and let you control interior and exterior lights from your car or from within the home to prevent you from tripping in the dark.

Suggested brand: Lutron AuroRa (888-588-7661, Lutron.com).

Cost: The AuroRa entry system starts at around $225 and provides wireless house lighting control for up to five dimmers that can be operated from the car or the bedside. Online retailers, such as Amazon.com offer it.

●**Create "wider" doorways.** Residential building codes and home builders don't consider the needs of older people who may need more than the standard 32-inch doorway, especially if they use a wheelchair or walker. Actually widening a doorway can be expensive and impractical, especially if it's along a weight-bearing wall.

Instead: Replace your standard door hinges with expandable "offset" hinges. These special hinges allow the door to close normally. But upon opening, they swing the door clear of the door frame by an extra two inches. This lets you use the entire width of the doorway when you enter or exit.

Cost: About $20 for a set of two door hinges. Available at home-improvement stores. A handy person can install these hinges because they fit in the existing holes in your door frame. Otherwise, a carpenter may charge about $100/hour.

•**Add a second handrail to staircases.** It's easier and safer to climb and descend when you can use both hands. Adding an extra handrail is an inexpensive and easy way to increase safety. Make sure both handrails are at the same height and between 30 and 34 inches above the front edge of the step. Also, for maximum safety, handrails should extend about six inches beyond the top and bottom steps if possible.

Cost: About $60 to $400 for each new handrail plus carpenter installation. Available at home-improvement stores.

•**Getting up from the couch.** Even young, healthy people can easily lose their balance when they stand up after being in a sitting position for a long time.

Solutions: Stand up slowly while grabbing on to the arm of the couch or chair before taking a step. If the arm isn't high enough to be of help, consider a CouchCane, a stabilizing device that adjusts in height from 29 to 32 inches.

Cost: About $100 at stores that sell wheelchairs, canes and other products for the physically impaired.

Kitchen

•**Lower your microwave.** Many home builders, contractors and home owners like to save space by mounting microwave ovens above the stove or high on a wall. This position is hazardous because it requires you to reach above your head to get hot foods or forces you to balance on a stool.

Better: If your existing microwave is on the wall, build a shelf under it where you can rest hot foods after they finish cooking. Or choose a new model with a tray feature that slides out and is easier to reach.

Example: The Sharp Insight Pro Microwave Drawer Oven installs just beneath your countertop. The entire oven slides open, drawer-style, giving you access to the cooking compartment from above.

Cost: About $1,500 for the microwave and $150 and up for carpenter installation. SharpUSA.com

•**Install a pullout kitchen faucet.** Lugging heavy pots of water to the stove can be difficult and even dangerous. Many plumbing manufacturers now offer kitchen faucets featuring high-arc, pullout spouts. You can remove the spout and use it as a sprayer hose to fill pots within three to five feet of the stove.

Cost: Starts at about $150 plus plumber installation. Available at home-improvement stores.

•**Install a pull-down shelving system inside your kitchen wall cabinets.** Top shelves in cabinets are difficult to reach. This simple device rests in your upper cabinet until you grab a handle on the shelf frame. A set of three or four shelves swings out of the cabinet and down toward you. The shelves lock in place so you can get the item you need.

Afterward, the whole unit swings back into place.

Suggested brand: Rev-A-Shelf's chrome pull-down shelving system for 24- and 36-inch cabinets. You can do the installation yourself.

Cost: $520 (800-626-1126, Rev-a-Shelf.com).

•**Kitchen tasks.** As we grow older, we often lose strength and agility, making it riskier to use knives and handle hot food.

For cutting food, consider semicircular cutting tools, such as the Rocking T Knife, that let you slice meat, bread and other foods by rocking the blade back and forth. Semicircular knives require less strength and are usually considered safer than standard butcher knives.

Cost: About $30 from kitchen appliance stores.

To make handling hot food easier, consider a "push-pull stick." These devices grip the oven rack so you can easily slide it in or out from a safe distance.

Cost: About $15 at kitchen speciality stores.

Bathroom

•**Add upscale grab bars near toilets and tubs.** Some people have avoided installing grab bars in their bathrooms because they look too institutional. Now, there are much more attractive versions. Brushed nickel or oil-rubbed bronze grab bars by Moen are designed to match other Moen bath accessories and faucets for a coordinated look. The grab bars meet all federal government guidelines. They have a stainless steel core and are 1¼ inches in diameter, making them easy to hold.

Cost: About $25 to $70 for the bar. Available at home-improvement stores. You can install them yourself, but it requires drilling holes in the wall.

Note: A towel bar is not the same thing as a grab bar—the latter is designed to be weight bearing and must be anchored into blocking (a secure mount). If they are in the right location, your contractor can attach grab bars to wall studs. Otherwise, a contractor can open the wall and install mounts for grab bars.

•**Elevated toilets.** At 17 to 19 inches high (a few inches higher than a standard toilet), "comfort height" or "chair height" toilets are often more comfortable for anyone to use, regardless of health condition. For people with painful joints or arthritis, they require less bending at the knee, and wheelchair users find them easier to get on and off of. They come in a range of designs, from utilitarian to trendy, and need not cost more than standard-height models.

CHAPTER 6

Secrets to Staying Steady On Your Feet

Fall-Proof Your Life

Mary Tinetti, MD, director of the Program on Aging and the Claude D. Pepper Older Americans Independence Center at the Yale School of Medicine in New Haven, Connecticut.

E very year in the US, about one-third of people age 65 and older fall, with 1.6 million treated in emergency rooms and 12,800 killed. But falling is not an inevitable result of aging.

Falling is associated with impairments (such as from stroke, gait or vision problems, or dementia) that are more common with age. But risk for falling is also increased by poor balance and muscle strength and by side effects of certain drugs, especially those prescribed for sleep and depression.

Risky Medications

Several types of widely prescribed drugs have been linked to an increased risk for falls, including...

•**Sleep medications,** such as the new generation of drugs heavily advertised on TV, including *eszopiclone* (Lunesta) and *zolpidem* (Ambien).

•**Antidepressants,** including selective serotonin reuptake inhibitors, such as *citalopram* (Celexa)...selective serotonin-norepinephrine reuptake inhibitors, such as *duloxetine* (Cymbalta)...and tricyclic antidepressants, such as *amitriptyline.*

•**Benzodiazepines** (antianxiety medications), such as *alprazolam* (Xanax).

•**Anticonvulsants,** such as *pregabalin* (Lyrica), a class of drugs that is prescribed not only for epilepsy but also for chronic pain problems, such as from nerve damage.

•**Atypical antipsychotics,** such as *quetiapine* (Seroquel), which are used to treat bipolar disorder…schizophrenia…and psychotic episodes (such as hallucinations) in people with dementia.

•**Blood pressure medications,** including diuretics, such as *furosamide* (Lasix)…and calcium channel blockers, such as *nifedipine* (Procardia).

Important: Taking five or more medications also is linked to an increased risk for falls.

Low Blood Pressure

Side effects of several medications (including drugs for Parkinson's disease, diuretics and heart drugs such as beta-blockers) may increase the risk of falling by causing postural hypotension (blood pressure drops when you stand up from lying down or sitting). Not enough blood flows to the heart to keep you alert and stable, and the body's normal mechanism to counteract this fails.

What to do: Ask your doctor to test you if you have symptoms, including feeling lightheaded or dizzy after standing. He/she will have you lie flat for five minutes, and then check your blood pressure immediately when you stand up. You will remain standing and have your pressure checked one or two minutes later. If systolic (top number) blood pressure drops at least 20 mmHg from lying to standing, you have postural hypotension.

If this is the case, ask about reducing your dosage of hypertensive, antidepressive and/or antipsychotic medications—the three drug types most likely to cause this condition.

Also: Drink more water—at least eight eight-ounce glasses a day. Dehydration can cause postural hypotension and is common among older people, who have a decreased sense of thirst.

Helpful: When you wake up in the morning, take your time getting out of bed. Sit on the edge of the bed for a few minutes while gently kicking forward with your lower legs and pumping your arms. This will move more blood to your heart and brain. Then stand up while holding on to a nearby stable object, such as a bedside table.

Vitamin D

Vitamin D promotes good muscle strength, so people with low blood levels of vitamin D may be at increased risk for falls. If your level is below 30 ng/mL, ask your doctor about taking a daily vitamin D supplement.

Guard Against Tumbles

Stephen Robinovitch, PhD, professor, kinesiology and engineering science, Simon Fraser University, British Columbia, Canada. His study was published in *The Lancet*.

You can fall at any age, of course, but the rate of falls during normal daily activities increases with age. So the older you get, the more careful you need to be. And age isn't the only risk factor—certain conditions also can play a role, such as vision impairment, cognitive problems and reduced muscle strength, to name just a few.

To help protect yourself (or a loved one) from taking a spill, focus on the number-one form of prevention, according to this study—try not to shift your center of gravity outside the base of support provided by your feet while moving around. *Here are some tips, which may help you avoid doing exactly that...*

● **When standing**—Keep your body weight evenly distributed between your feet—don't lean too far sideways or on the heels or balls of your feet.

● **When walking**—Avoid abrupt turns—turn slowly, with your whole body at once (don't swivel your head and torso around without moving your lower half, too, for instance).

● **When reaching**—Instead of grasping for high items that are near the limit of your reach (such as the door of a kitchen cabinet that's above the refrigerator) and causing your body to lurch awkwardly, use a wide, low step stool or call someone taller to help.

● **When bending**—If you've dropped, say, your car keys, instead of leaning down with your upper body while keeping your legs straight (which causes your center of gravity to shift forward), lower yourself by bending your knees and moving into a squatting position.

Keep an Eye on Pets Below

Pets cause more than 86,000 people to fall and injure themselves each year. The main causes are tripping over the animals or being pulled or pushed by them. Dogs are responsible for 88% of the injuries, and often the most severe ones. Most accidents occur in the home. Children age 14 and younger and adults ages 35 to 54 are the most likely to get hurt.

Self-defense: Be aware of fall hazards caused by pets, and have dogs professionally trained.

Centers for Disease Control and Prevention, Atlanta.

Catch Your Balance Problem Before It's Too Late

Jason Jackson, MSPT, a physical therapist in the outpatient rehabilitation department at Mount Sinai Hospital in New York City, where he specializes in balance training, along with prosthetic training, manual therapy and neuromuscular disease.

N
o one expects to get seriously injured—or even die—from a fall. But it happens all the time. And while older adults are at greatest risk for falls, there are no age requirements for taking a tumble.

Surprising statistic: Even among adults in their 30s, 40s and 50s, falls are the leading cause of nonfatal injuries (more than 3 million each year) that are treated in US hospital emergency departments. For adults age 65 and older, falls are the leading cause of fatal injuries.

Certain "fall hazards" are well known—electrical cords and area rugs… slippery floors…medications such as sleeping pills and blood pressure drugs… vision problems…and even poorly fitting shoes.

What often gets overlooked: Subtle changes in the neuromuscular system (the nervous system and muscles working together), which helps keep us upright. Regardless of your age, exercising and strengthening this system before you get unsteady (or fall) is one of the best steps you can take to protect your health. *Here's how…*

Why Our Balance Slips

Does your foot or ankle feel a little wobbly when you stand on one leg? Some of that is probably due to diminished strength and flexibility. After about age 40, we begin to lose roughly 1% of our muscle mass every year. As we age, we also become more sedentary and less flexible. These factors make the body less able to adapt to and correct a loss of balance.

The nervous system also gets less sensitive with age.

Example: Sensory receptors known as proprioceptors are found in the nerve endings of muscles, tendons, joints and the inner ear. These receptors make us aware of our bodies in space (proprioception) and can detect even the slightest variations in body positions and movements. But they don't work well in people who don't exercise them (see suggestions on next page)—and these people find it harder to keep their balance.

The other danger: Muscle weakness, even when it's slight, can lead to apprehension about losing your balance. You might then start to avoid physical activities that you feel are risky—walking on uneven pavement, for example. But avoiding such challenges to your balance actually accelerates both muscle and nervous system declines.

Are You Steady?

If you're afraid of falling or have a history of falls, a professional balance assessment, done by your doctor or a physical therapist, is the best way to find out how steady you are on your feet. The assessment usually includes tests such as the following (don't try these tests on your own if you feel unsteady)...

•**Sit-to-stand.** Sit in a straight-backed chair. If your balance and leg strength are good, you'll be able to stand up without pushing off with your hands.

•**Stand with your feet touching.** You should be able to hold this position for 15 seconds without any wobbling.

•**The nudge test.** Ask someone to gently push on your hip while you're in a normal stance. If you stagger or throw out your hands to catch yourself, your balance is questionable. If you start to fall, your balance needs improvement.

Boost Your Balance

Balance, like strength and endurance, can be improved with simple workouts. Incorporate the exercises below into your daily routine—while at the grocery store, in the office, while watching TV, etc. Do them for about 15 minutes to 30 minutes a day, three to four days a week (daily if you have the time). *What to do...* *

•**One-legged stands.** You don't have to set aside time to do this exercise. You simply stand on one leg as you go about your daily activities—while waiting in line, for example. Lift your foot about six inches to 12 inches off the floor to the front, side and back. Try to hold each position for about 15 seconds, then switch legs. This strengthens the muscles in the ankles, hips and knees—all of which play a key role in one's balance.

•**Heel raises.** This move is good for balance and strength. While standing, rise up on your toes as far as you can. Drop back to the starting position, then

---

*Do these exercises next to a stable object, such as a countertop, if you feel unsteady. Also, they are more easily done while wearing shoes. When you feel comfortable doing these moves, you can perform them barefoot to add difficulty.

do it again. Try for 10 repetitions. You can make this exercise more difficult by holding weights. Start with three-pound weights, gradually increasing weight as you build tolerance.

For More Benefits

Once you have become comfortable with the exercises described earlier, you can up your game with the following to keep you even safer from falling...

●**Balance on a Bosu ball.** It's a rubber-like half-ball (about two feet in diameter) that you can use for dozens of at-home workouts, including balance and abdominal exercises.

Cost: About $100, on Amazon.com and in some sporting-goods stores.

Example: With the flat side on the floor, start by standing with both feet on the ball. Your muscles and joints will make hundreds of small adjustments to keep you balanced. When you get better at it, try to stand on one leg on the ball. When you're really comfortable, have someone toss you a basketball or tennis ball while you maintain your balance.

Urinary Problems Are a Hidden Fall Danger

In a recent four-year study of 5,872 men (age 65 or older), those who reported moderate lower urinary tract problems, such as urgency to urinate or urinary frequency, were 21% more likely to fall at least twice within a one-year period than those without urinary problems.

Theory: Falls may occur when a man is rushing to the bathroom—during the day or at night.

If you have urinary tract symptoms: Ask your doctor about treatment.

J. Kellogg Parsons, MD, assistant professor of surgery, Cancer Prevention & Control Program, Moores Cancer Center, University of California, San Diego.

Just for Fun

You don't always need formal balance exercises. *Try this...*

●**Walk barefoot.** Most of us spend our days in well-padded shoes that minimize the "feedback" between our feet and the ground. Walking without shoes for at least a few minutes each day strengthens the intrinsic muscles in the feet and improves stability. If you prefer to wear socks, be sure to use nonslip varieties that have treads to avoid slipping on wood or tiled floors.

Also helpful: Minimalist walking/running shoes. They're made by most major footwear companies, such as New Balance, Adidas and Nike, as well as by Vivobarefoot. Because they have a minimal amount of heel cushioning and arch support, they give the same benefits as barefoot walking but with a little extra protection.

•**Do these exercises next to a stable object, such as a countertop, if you feel unsteady.** Also, they are more easily done while wearing shoes. When you feel comfortable doing these moves, you can perform them barefoot to add difficulty.

Way Beyond Calcium: Minerals Your Bones Need Most

Mao Shing Ni, PhD, DOM (doctor of oriental medicine), **LAc** (licensed acupuncturist), is chancellor and cofounder of Yo San University in Los Angeles and codirector of Tao of Wellness, an acupuncture and Chinese medicine clinic in Santa Monica, California. He is author of *Secrets of Longevity: Hundreds of Ways to Live to Be 100.* TaoOfWellness.com

A recent study has us worried that getting too much calcium from supplements increases our risk for heart attacks. That's why many of us are cutting back on calcium supplements to protect our hearts… and, hopefully, boosting our consumption of calcium-rich foods (which are not linked to cardiovascular problems), such as dairy products and dark green leafy vegetables, to protect our bones.

But: This makes it more important than ever to guard against osteoporosis. An excellent strategy is to be sure to get enough of four other essential, yet less familiar, minerals that our bones need to stay strong. These minerals are especially vital for women, who are four times more likely than men to develop osteoporosis.

> ## Men Get Osteoporosis, Too!
>
> Up to one in four men over age 50 will break a bone due to osteoporosis.
>
> *Problem:* A recent analysis that looked at 439 patients' medical records found that men are less likely than women to be screened for osteoporosis and far less likely to be treated for the condition after a fracture.
>
> *Why it matters:* Treating the fracture but not the underlying cause puts patients at risk for future breaks.
>
> Tamara D. Rozental, MD, associate professor of orthopedic surgery, Harvard Medical School, Boston.

The ideal way to get these minerals is through food because foods contain complementary components that enhance nutrient absorption. For a mineral-rich, bone-building diet, follow the guidelines below. For serving sizes, see "Amounts that constitute one serving of…" at the end of this article.

Boron helps the body use calcium, vitamin D and other nutrients vital to bone formation.

Be sure to eat: At least three servings per day of nuts (almonds, hazelnuts, peanuts) or nut butters...or fruits (apples, avocados, bananas, grapes, oranges, pears, tangelos).

Added boost: Dried fruits are especially rich in boron—but don't overdo it on these, as they also are high in sugar. Onions are another good source.

Manganese is essential for the proper formation and maintenance of bone, cartilage and connective tissue.

Be sure to eat: Two or more daily servings of legumes (chickpeas, lentils, lima beans)...nuts (chestnuts, hazelnuts, pecans, pine nuts)...or whole grains (barley, brown rice, bulgur, couscous, oats).

Added boost: For extra manganese, have some pineapple, blackberries, raspberries or strawberries.

Silicon assists calcium with bone growth and increases collagen, the protein component of bones. A study published in the *Journal of Bone and Mineral Research* showed that silicon was particularly helpful for premenopausal women.

Be sure to eat: Four or more servings per week of whole grains (barley, brown rice, oats)...or fruits (apples, bananas, cherries, grapes, mangoes, pineapples, plums).

Added boost: Silicon also is found in cabbage, celery, cucumbers, green beans and tofu.

Zinc produces enzymes that recycle worn-out portions of bone protein and help heal injured bones.

Be sure to eat: Two servings a week of shellfish (crabs, lobster, oysters)...lean meat (beef, lamb, pork, veal)...poultry (chicken, duck, turkey)...legumes (black-eyed peas, chickpeas, lentils, lima beans, navy beans)...or seeds (pumpkin, sesame, squash, sunflower).

Added boost: Other good sources include barley, bulgur, cashews, pine nuts, ricotta cheese and yogurt.

Amounts that constitute one serving of…

- **Fish, meat, poultry or a soy product**—Three to four ounces.
- **Cooked grains or whole-grain cereal**—One-half cup…or one slice of whole-grain bread.

- **Chopped raw or cooked vegetables or legumes**—One-half cup.

- **Fruit**—One whole small fruit…one-half cup of berries or diced fruit…or one-quarter cup of dried fruit.

- **Nuts or seeds**—Two ounces…or one tablespoon of peanut butter or other nut butter.

Potassium—The Mineral Calcium Needs to Keep Your Bones Strong

Janet Brill, PhD, RDN, dietitian and fitness expert, Allentown, Pennsylvania. She is author of *Blood Pressure Down: The 10-Step Plan to Lower Your Blood Pressure in 4 Weeks Without Prescription Drugs* and *Cholesterol Down: Take Control of Your Cholesterol—Without Drugs*. DrJanet.com

You've probably been led to believe that if you just drink enough milk, eat enough yogurt and cheese, get some broccoli and maybe take a calcium supplement, you will be assured of having healthy bones that are resistant to osteoporosis. Wrong! The truth is, if you're not getting enough of another essential nutrient, potassium, you won't get the benefit from all that calcium. *Here's how to make sure you get the amount of potassium you really need for healthy bones…*

It's Not About Calcium Anymore

With all the constant hoopla about calcium, you would never guess that numerous studies have shown that potassium is just as important for bone health. So why does calcium get all the publicity? Maybe even doctors don't realize how important potassium is…and maybe the supplement industry is just too hooked on its calcium profits to put the spotlight somewhere else. But the fact is, a lot of people who think they're doing good for their bones are consuming too little potassium. And their bones are suffering for it.

Strong proof of the importance of potassium: Researchers recently analyzed 14 high-quality studies on the effects of potassium supplements on

Vitamin K Strengthens Bones

Vitamin K strengthens bones. Older people who consumed the most broccoli, spinach and other leafy green vegetables rich in vitamin K had higher bone mineral density than those who consumed the least vitamin K. Supplements of vitamin K also improve bone quality, but it is best to get the vitamin from food sources, which have other nutrients as well.

Caution: If you are taking a blood-thinning medication, such as warfarin, talk to your doctor before increasing your intake of vitamin K.

Study of 365 people by researchers at Universitat Rovira i Virgili, Reus, Spain, published in *Bone*.

bone health and found that people who had higher intakes of potassium excreted less calcium in their urine and had markers in their blood that showed less bone loss. The reason? Potassium aids calcium absorption.

Thus, diets higher in potassium might be a way to improve bone strength and help prevent bone weakening and osteoporosis.

Potassium has been shown to slow down a process called bone resorption, which happens in our bodies all the time as a natural process. In the bone-resorption process, small cells called osteoclasts break down bone to make room for new bone growth. However, as we age, new bone formation slows down and can be outpaced by bone resorption. The result is thin and brittle bones that can easily fracture.

High intake of potassium has been shown to significantly reduce the excretion of calcium in the urine. Furthermore, potassium neutralizes the excess acid from the metabolism of a heavy meat-eating diet.

Aim to get 4,700 milligrams (mg) of potassium a day, an amount in line with the recommendation of the Institute of Medicine of the National Academy of Sciences, which helps set US health policy. Stay away from potassium supplements, which do not deliver nutrition as efficiently as nutrition-rich food. Besides, potassium supplements can cause intestinal problems such as diarrhea, stomach upset and flatulence in some people.

And people on diuretics or other blood pressure medications and those with kidney disease need to be extra cautious about potassium supplementation. Certain diuretics, such as Aldactone, Midamor and Dyrenium, and many other blood pressure medications, such as Avapro, Cozaar, Diovan and Vasotec, and also NSAIDs, when taken with potassium supplements can lead to potassium excess in the body. This condition, called hyperkalemia, can cause symptoms of tingling extremities, muscle weakness or irregular heart beat that can result in cardiac arrest. If you're taking any medication, particularly the ones mentioned above, it is strongly advised that you don't take a potassium supplement without first consulting an MD or a naturopathic doctor.

Finding Potassium in Your Food

So where does safe, natural potassium come from? Think 'P' for potassium and produce.

Of course not all produce is created equal. Some is more chock-full of potassium than others. In addition to the best-known potassium sources—bananas and white potatoes—a "hot list" of high-potassium foods might include spinach, kale, beet greens (and other dark, leafy green vegetables), cantaloupe, kidney beans and avocado.

Stop Flushing Your Calcium Down the Drain

Elson M. Haas, MD, founder and director of the Preventive Medical Center of Marin in San Rafael, California. He also is the author of numerous books, including Staying Healthy with Nutrition: The Complete Guide to Diet and Nutritional Medicine. PMCMarin. com

Are you conscientiously eating calcium-rich foods and following your doctor's orders about calcium supplement use? That's good—but not good enough to ensure that your bones benefit.

Reason: Some foods contain substances that interfere with calcium absorption, so whatever else you eat along with your calcium influences how much of the mineral goes to your bones…and how much literally gets flushed away when you go to the bathroom.

To tip this balance in your favor, it helps to allow a few hours to elapse between eating the foods that you rely on for calcium and eating the types of foods that reduce calcium absorption, So just what kinds of foods are we talking about?

Calcium-rich foods: These include beans (great northern, navy, white)…Chinese cabbage…dairy products…fortified cereals… leafy greens (beet greens, collards, dandelion greens, kale, turnip greens)…nuts… okra…rice…seafood (crab, salmon, ocean perch, sardines, shrimp)…seeds…and soy products.

DHEA Supplements Build Better Bones

Older women (not men) who supplemented daily with the hormone dehydroepiandrosterone (DHEA) plus calcium and vitamin D had a 4% average increase in spinal bone density after two years—enough to reduce spinal fracture risk by up to 50%. Women who took only calcium and vitamin D had no bone density increase. Ask your doctor about taking 50 mg of DHEA daily. Avoid DHEA if you have a history of breast or endometrial cancer.

Edward Weiss, PhD, associate professor of nutrition and dietetics, Doisy College of Health Sciences, Saint Louis University.

Here's what interferes with calcium...

•**Sodium.** When you eat too much sodium, the excess is excreted in your urine—but when that sodium leaves your body, it drags calcium with it.

Best: Limit daily consumption of sodium to no more than 2,300 mg or about the amount in one teaspoon of salt. What if you do go overboard on salt? Potassium helps limit sodium-induced calcium excretion, so have a high-potassium food (banana, cantaloupe) with your calcium.

•**Caffeine.** Do you often have calcium-rich yogurt for breakfast or take your calcium pill with your morning meal—then wash it down with a big mug of coffee or tea? Caffeine from any source works against strong bones by interfering with calcium absorption and causing more of the mineral to be lost through the urine.

Better: Have your morning yogurt with a glass of orange juice instead, since its vitamin C and magnesium improve calcium absorption...or take your supplement in the afternoon or evening, after you've finished drinking coffee for the day.

•**Phytates.** Found in high-fiber foods such as berries, corn, nuts, oatmeal, rye and especially wheat bran, phytates are substances that bind calcium, reducing its absorption. Fiber-rich foods have many health benefits, so of course you don't want to shun them...but if you're increasing your fiber intake (for instance, to help regulate digestion), be sure to increase your calcium intake, too.

•**Phosphorus.** This mineral, which is plentiful in meat and poultry, has many important functions in the body. But for proper bone density, a delicate balance must be maintained between phosphorus and calcium—which means that as phosphorus intake increases, the need for calcium increases, too.

Problem: Ideally, people should eat more calcium than phosphorus, but the typical meat-focused Western diet contains roughly two to four times more phosphorus than calcium. Also, because both phosphorus and calcium require vitamin D for absorption, phosphorus-rich foods compete with calcium-rich foods for the available vitamin D.

Bone smart: Ask your doctor about supplementing with vitamin D. Also, cut back on meat and focus more on plant foods...and be aware that carbonated beverages such as colas have as much as 500 mg of phosphorus in one serving—so say "so long" to soda.

Nighttime note: Has your doctor recommended calcium supplements? Choose a brand that also includes magnesium for maximum absorption... and take half of your daily dose at bedtime—it may even help you relax and sleep better.

Yoga for Bone Health

Carol Krucoff is a yoga therapist at Duke Integrative Medicine, which is part of the Duke University Health System in Durham, North Carolina (HealingMoves.com). She is author of *Healing Yoga for Neck and Shoulder Pain* and the DVD *Relax into Yoga: Finding Ease in Body and Mind*.

If yoga makes you think of stretching and improving your flexibility, think again. The ancient practice of yoga actually has something in common with walking, running, dancing and weight training—all are weight-bearing exercises. So, if you need to do weight-bearing exercises to protect your bones, consider yoga—especially if you don't have access to weights or want a form of exercise that's easier on your joints than an activity like running. Specific yoga poses can help improve bone strength and general endurance.

One of the benefits of yoga for bone health: Many yoga positions require that you support your body weight with your legs and/or arms. In some positions, such as downward dog or plank, both your arms and legs support your body weight. These postures provide a boost to bones in both the upper and lower body, a claim that can't be made by activities such as running or walking, which just involve the lower body. A recent study by researchers at University of California at Los Angeles found that yoga reduced the curvature of the spine in adults with hyperkyphosis (also known as "dowager's hump), a condition that often is caused by bone loss. Another study by researchers based in Bangkok found that postmenopausal women who practiced yoga had significantly lower levels of bone degradation than those who didn't practice yoga.

Here are a few simple yoga poses that help to build bones. For best results, do each pose three times a week. (For details on how long to hold each pose, see below.)

Bone-building yoga poses…

Chair Pose

What it does: Strengthens the bones of the legs and hips.

How to do it: Stand with feet hip-distance apart. Extend your arms forward at shoulder height. (To make the move more difficult, you can put your arms over your head with your upper arms parallel to your ears.) Bend your knees, bow forward at the hips, stick your bottom out and lower it down as if you were going to sit in an invisible chair. Make sure that your back is straight, not rounded, and that your knees are not in front of your toes. Hold the position for two or three slow, deep breaths, then return to standing. Repeat five times, working your way up to 10 times.

Spinal Balance

What it does: Strengthens bones in the arms, shoulders and thighs.

How to do it: Come onto all fours—with your knees directly under your hips and your wrists directly under your shoulders. Moving slowly, extend the left leg out behind you and raise it to hip height, toes toward the floor. Next, extend your right arm forward and raise it to shoulder height. Hold for one full, easy breath. Then return to the starting position and switch sides. Repeat three times on each side, working up to holding the pose each time for three breaths.

Warrior II

What it does: Strengthens bones of the lower body.

How to do it: Step your feet about three to four feet apart. Extend your arms out to both sides and parallel to the floor, palms facing down. Turn your left foot 90 degrees to the left and angle the toes of your right foot toward the left. Bend your left knee (make sure that your left knee is over your left ankle) and align the arch of your right foot with the heel of your left foot. Straighten your right leg, pressing the outer heel into the floor. Gaze out over the left fingertips. Hold for three to five breaths, then switch sides and repeat.

Plank

What it does: Strengthens bones in the arms, shoulders and legs.

How to do it: Come onto all fours with your palms flat against the floor under your shoulders, fingers spread wide. Extend your right leg out behind you, toes tucked under. Next, extend your left leg out behind you, toes tucked under, so that your body forms a straight line from the top of your head to your heels. Stay here, balanced on your hands and toes, for three full breaths. If you can't breathe easily with your legs straight, bring your knees to the floor and perform the pose with your knees on the floor. This version of the pose is easier to do but still strengthens the arm bones.

When starting any new physical activity, including yoga, it's a good idea to speak to your doctor to ensure that it is safe for you. To learn the postures accurately, you can take a class with a registered teacher. The Yoga Alliance (YogaAlliance.org), a national yoga education organization, which maintains a national registry of teachers who have completed at least 200 hours of yoga teacher training, can help you find a teacher in your area.

How to Fall Down: Tricks from an Oscar-Winning Stuntman

Hal Needham, who appeared as a stuntman in more than 4,000 television episodes and more than 300 feature films. He is author of *Stuntman! My Car-Crashing, Plane-Jumping, Bone-Breaking, Death-Defying Hollywood Life*.

When we fall, our natural instinct is to reach out for the ground with our hands. Unfortunately, that only increases our odds of injury—our hands, wrists and arms are full of small bones that are easily broken. *Instead, when you realize you are falling...*

1. Buckle your knees. This can in essence lower the height that your upper body falls by as much as a foot or two, significantly reducing the impact when you hit the ground. In a forward fall, it might result in bruised knees, but that's better than a broken bone in the upper body.

Helpful: In a backward fall, tuck your head into your chest as you buckle your knees—try to turn yourself into a ball.

2. Throw one arm across your chest whether you're falling forward or backward. Do this with enough force that it turns your body to one side. It doesn't matter which arm you use.

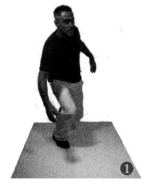 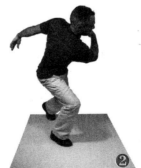 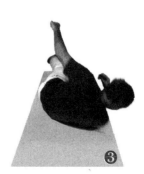

3. Rotate the rest of your body in the direction that you threw your arm, increasing your spin. If you can rotate enough, you can come down mainly on your backside, a well-padded part of the body unlikely to experience a serious injury.

Trouble is, while stuntmen know exactly when and where they're going to fall, real-world falls usually take people by surprise. It can be difficult to overcome instinct and put this falling strategy into action in the split second before hitting the ground.

Practice can help. If you have access to a thick gym mat and you don't have health issues that make it risky, try out this falling technique until it feels natural.

CHAPTER 7

Drive Safer Longer

You Don't Have to Give Up Those Car Keys

Patrick Baker, an occupational therapist, certified low-vision therapist and certified driver-rehabilitation specialist at the Cleveland Clinic in Cleveland, Ohio.

Richard A. Marottoli, MD, associate professor of medicine at Yale School of Medicine and medical director of the Dorothy Adler Geriatric Assessment Center at Yale-New Haven Hospital, both in New Haven, Connecticut.

D riving may be the most hazardous thing that most of us do each day, but simply growing older—or having a chronic medical condition, no matter what your age, that affects your vision, thought process or physical abilities—doesn't mean that you can't continue to be independent.

To drive safely as long as possible: It's crucial to proactively avoid problems that can limit your car-handling competence. *Here's how...*

Preempt Problems

Beyond commonsense imperatives such as getting regular medical, vision and hearing checkups, a few simple steps will help ensure that your driving abilities are intact.

At your checkup with your primary care doctor, have a candid talk to discuss any medical conditions you may have that could affect your driving now or in the future.

For example, a stroke may result in lingering visual or movement problems...diabetes might be causing neuropathy in your feet, making it difficult to feel the gas or brake pedals...and cataracts, macular degeneration or glaucoma may limit vision if it's not carefully treated. A conversation with your doctor can help you minimize these issues and prevent them from becoming a bigger problem down the road. *Also…*

Manage Your Meds

Some prescription or over-the-counter medications can impair your ability to drive by triggering drowsiness, cutting concentration, inducing shakiness or uncoordinated movements, or increasing your reaction time. Taking multiple drugs—a common practice among older adults and those coping with chronic medical problems—can make matters even worse by amplifying medication side effects. Certain dietary supplements, such as melatonin or valerian, may also have an effect.

What to find out: Show your doctor or pharmacist a list of all the medications (prescription and over-the-counter) and dietary supplements you take and ask how they interact and may affect your driving abilities.

Also: Ask if the timing of when you take any drugs or supplements that may affect cognition or coordination can be altered—for example, taken before bedtime instead of in the morning.

Important: If you are on painkillers or narcotics, also ask your spouse or a trusted friend if the medication makes you "loopy"—an effect that you may not notice but is perhaps obvious to another person.

Customize Your Car

Age can compromise your eyesight and bring physical changes that make it more difficult to see the road while driving—for example, many people lose one to three inches of height due to bone loss and spinal compression. Or a stroke or eye condition (such as cataracts) may affect your peripheral vision, interfering with your ability to spot traffic alongside your car. To address these changes, it helps to customize your car. *Here's how…*

• **Set power seats at the highest level.** Also, consider adding a firm cushion (such as the durable type used for outdoor furniture) to the driver's seat so that your chin is at least three inches higher than the top of the steering wheel.

• **Use extra (or bigger) mirrors inside and/or outside your car to increase your field of vision.** For example, you can get a mirror that attaches to your rearview mirror to expand your view to the rear. Or you can get bigger mirrors or extra mirrors that can be bolted onto existing side mirrors or the side of the car itself. Check with your car dealer for details for your make and model.

•**Keep your headlights clean.** Also, consider replacing the bulbs—even before they burn out. The bulbs get dimmer before they've completely burned out.

•**Opt for automatic.** If you're buying a new car, be sure to get one with automatic transmission, power steering and power brakes, which don't require as much strength to operate. Also, consider a car with backup alert sensors, which detect objects in your blind spots.

Spruce Up Your Skills

A driving refresher course (ideally taken every three to five years) will keep you up to date on the newest traffic rules and can reduce road mishaps.

Good news: Some car insurance companies even lower premium rates if you take one of these courses, which usually lasts four to eight hours.

Good choice: A course such as those offered by AAA or AARP is likely to have an instructor who is well versed in issues facing older adults—as well as classmates who are true peers. If you are interested in taking a driver course because of a medical condition, consult The Association for Driver Rehabilitation Specialists (ADED.net and search "CDRS provider") to find a program near you. *Avoid dangerous situations…*

•**Use routes that minimize left turns**—they are more dangerous than right turns. When waiting to turn left, keep your wheels straight so you won't be pushed into oncoming traffic if hit from behind.

•**On the highway, stay in the right lane whenever possible.** There's less risk of being tailgated, and you probably won't need to change lanes to exit.

•**Minimize travel on congested or poorly lit roads.**

•**Do not drive in rain or snow or when you feel tired or stressed.** Stay home or call a taxi.

See and Be Seen

•**To determine if you're tailgating,** pick a spot that the car in front of you passes, then count the seconds until you reach that spot. If it's less than three seconds—or six seconds in rain or fog—back off.

•**Use your window defroster on high heat** to clear window fog quickly… then switch to cool air (not cold) to keep fog from coming back. This works in all weather.

•**Keep your windows clean inside and outside.**

●**Be on the watch for distracted drivers.** Stay focused yourself, too—don't talk on the phone or eat or fiddle with the CD player or have emotional conversations with your passengers.

●**Keep headlights on, even during the day**—it makes you more visible to others. Clean headlights often.

●**If you have poor night vision, drive only in daylight.**

Master New Car Technology

●**Put your seat as far back as you comfortably can to avoid being injured by the air bag if it deploys.**

●**Tilt the steering wheel so that the air bag points toward your chest, not your head.** If your steering wheel telescopes, move it closer to the dashboard to lessen air bag impact.

●**If you skid, do not "pump" anti-lock brakes**—just brake steadily.

Focus on Footwear

When it comes to hitting the gas and brake, what's on our feet can be just as important as our ability to see and react. *Consider these important footwear-related issues...*

●**Choose the right sneaker.** Running-style sneakers with soles that are thick, chunky and/or beveled can catch on pedals as you move your foot, so opt for a flat sole, such as a tennis-style or walking sneaker.

●**Go for thin soles.** People with diabetic neuropathy or limited foot sensation should wear thinner-soled shoes while driving. Thin soles, which don't have much padding between the bottom of the feet and the car pedals, give you a better sense of how hard you are pushing the brake and accelerator.

Important: Be sure to choose a car that "fits" you well—with good sight lines to the sides and rear...controls that are easy to reach...and a model that is easy for you to get in and out of.

Over 50? These Gadgets Make Driving Safer, Easier...and More Fun

Jim Miller, an advocate for senior citizens, writes "Savvy Senior," a weekly information column syndicated in more than 400 newspapers nationwide. Based in Norman, Oklahoma, he also offers a free senior news service at SavvySenior.org.

While age doesn't make someone a bad driver, it typically does bring about physical and cognitive changes that can make driving more challenging. Fortunately, to help keep aging drivers safe, there is a wide variety of affordable devices and tools that you can purchase today and add to your vehicle to help with many different needs.

Entry and Exit

Each year in the US, an estimated 37,000 seniors are injured simply entering or exiting vehicles. *If a mobility problem or limited range of motion is hampering your ability to get in and out of your auto, here are some items that can help...*

•**Metro Car Handle** is a small portable support handle (made of steel with a nonslip grip for your hand) that inserts into the U-shaped hooklike striker plate on the door frame. (The striker plate is the piece of metal that holds the door closed in the event of a side collision.) $29* 800-506-9901, Stander.com.

•**CarCaddie Mobility Aid** is a nylon handle that hooks around the top of the door window frame. $10. 800-506-9901, Stander.com.

•**Swivel Seat Cushion** is a round portable pad that turns 360 degrees to help drivers and passengers rotate into and out of a vehicle. Works best on flat car seats. $23. 800-506-9901, Stander.com.

Vision Helpers

Many older drivers are especially sensitive to glare and/or have difficulty turning to look over their shoulders. *Products that can help...*

•**Glare Guard Polarized Sun Visor is a plastic tinted visor that clips onto your existing sun visor to remove sun glare without obstructing vision.** It also incorporates a sliding shield that lets you further block extra-bright glare spots. $30. Amazon.com.

*Prices subject to change.

•**Wireless Back-up Camera System** is a small camera with night vision that attaches to your rear license plate so that you can see what's behind you without turning around. It comes with a 7-inch LCD color monitor that mounts to your dash or windshield. $79. Amazon.com.

Arthritic Hands

Drivers who have arthritic or weak hands may find turning the ignition key, twisting open the gas cap, and other tasks difficult. *Tools that can help…*

•**Hole In One Key Holder.** For $30, this plastic handle device attaches to car keys to provide additional leverage when turning the key in the ignition. Or for car keys with thick plastic head covers, there's a Key Lever for $35. 888-940-0605, LiveOakMed.com.

•**Gas Cap Grip.** To help at the pump, this long-handled device fits onto most gas caps and works like a wrench to help open the gas tank with ease. $10. 855-202-7394, MilesKimball.com.

Small Drivers

Most people shrink a little as they get older…and for those who were small to start with, it can be difficult to see over the steering wheel or to reach a vehicle's pedals without being too close to the airbag. *Solutions include…*

•**Ortho Wedge Cushion.** This seat cushion supports the back and elevates you a few extra inches to help you see. $15. 800-231-5806, Wagan.com.

•**Foot pedal extensions** allow you to reach the pedals while keeping you 10 to 12 inches from the steering wheel. Costs for a gas and brake pedal range from $128 to $220, depending on length. They should be installed by a mechanic to ensure safety. 888-372-0153, PedalExtenders.com.

Seat Belt Aids

Products that help enhance seat belt comfort and functionality without sacrificing safety…

•**Easy Reach Seat Belt Handle** is a six-inch rubber extension handle that attaches to your seat belt strap to make it easier to reach. $18. 888-940-0605, LiveOakMed.com.

•**Zento Deals Seatbelt Shoulder Pad** fits around the shoulder strap to protect your neck and shoulder from rubbing and chafing. $9. Amazon.com.

•**Seat Belt Adjuster.** This small plastic clip, which attaches to the shoulder strap and lap belt, allows you to adjust the seat belt shoulder strap between shoulder and neck for greater comfort and safety. $7 for a set of two. 855-202-7391, EasyComforts.com.

Night Driving Strategies

William Van Tassel, PhD, manager of driver-training operations at AAA's national office in Heathrow, Florida. He holds a doctorate in safety education. AAA.com

Fatal car crashes are three times more likely at night than during the day, per mile driven. The dark makes it more difficult to spot trouble on the road, and the late hour makes it more likely that we share the road with drunk or drowsy drivers.

Older drivers in particular often have trouble at night. Our eyes' ability to see in limited light declines steadily starting in our 30s. This happens so gradually that many older drivers don't realize how much night vision they have lost.

Fortunately, minor adjustments to our driving habits and vehicles can make a major difference in our night time driving risks. *Five things drivers can do to see and drive better at night...*

•**Shift your gaze down and to the right to avoid being blinded by approaching headlights.** Use the edge of the road or the line marking the outside of your lane as a reference point until the headlights have passed.

If you are blinded by oncoming headlights, drive conservatively until your eyes readjust to low light—that typically takes around six seconds—but resist the urge to brake if there are cars close behind you. The drivers behind you might have been temporarily blinded by the oncoming headlights, too, and not notice that you've slowed.

•**Increase your following distance.** In clear daytime conditions, three seconds is considered a safe following distance—pick a fixed object along the roadside and count off the seconds from when the car in front of you passes it until you do. At night, five or six seconds is more appropriate, since, among other things, our reaction times are slowed if we're drowsy.

•**Check your mirrors frequently.** This increases your awareness of what's happening outside the beams of light cast by your headlights. It also keeps your mind active and attentive while you are driving.

Also: Avoid using cruise control after dark, and alter your speed periodically. This, too, keeps the brain more engaged, combating drowsiness.

•**Tap your brakes a few times before stopping if there are cars behind you.** This makes your brake lights flash—and flashing lights grab the attention of drowsy or drunk drivers much better than steady lights.

Also: Use your blinkers well before you slow to turn. Use your hazard lights if you must stop on the side of a dark road.

•**If you wear glasses, choose ones that have an anti-reflective (AR) coating.** This clear coating cuts down on lens glare, improving your ability to see at night despite oncoming headlights.

Automotive Adjustments

Five ways to prep your car for safer night driving...

•**Adjust your side mirrors so that you can almost, but not quite, see the outside of your own car in them.** Most drivers angle their side mirrors a bit too far to the inside, which allows the headlights of vehicles behind them to reflect into their eyes, reducing their night vision. Side mirrors angled too far inside also increase drivers' "blind spots" behind and to the side of the car at night and during the day.

Also, don't forget to switch your center rearview mirror to its night setting after dark to avoid headlights reflecting into your eyes. If your car has a self-dimming rearview mirror, double-check to make sure this function is turned on and working.

•**Clean your windshield, windows, headlights and taillights frequently.** Windshield and window smudges and grime that are barely noticeable during the day can cause tremendous glare when hit by other vehicles' headlights at night. Remember to clean the inside of the glass, not just the outside.

Dirt also builds up on headlights and taillights, dramatically reducing their brightness over time.

Consider installing enhanced replacement headlight bulbs on your car. These may help you see more of the road ahead for perhaps just $10 or $20 extra per bulb.

•**Dim your interior gauges slightly.** The glow from a bright dashboard can detract from your eyes' ability to see outside the vehicle at night. Turn gauge brightness down a bit, even if this means that you must strain a little to read the gauges—seeing what's outside your car is more important than reading dashboard gauges. Also, don't allow any passengers to have lights on inside the car when you're driving.

•**Turn on your headlights at dusk, or use them all the time.** Headlights won't provide much help seeing the road until it's quite dark—but they do help other drivers see you at all hours, which reduces the odds of collisions.

Using your high-beam headlights can further improve your vision at night. Just be sure to dim them when you detect another vehicle, either coming toward you or traveling ahead of you in the same direction.

Drugs That Increase the Risk for Car Crashes

Hui-Ju Tsai, MPH, PhD, associate investigator, division of biostatistics and bioinformatics, Institute of Population Health Sciences, National Health Research Institutes, Taiwan. She is lead author of a study published in *British Journal of Pharmacology*.

I f you are among the millions of people taking any of these drugs, then you'll definitely want to know whether or not you're at increased risk...

Which Drugs Were Studied?

Researchers looked at two groups of data on people age 18 or over. One group was made up of people who had a record of being in a car accident (as a driver, not a passenger) at some point over a recent 10-year span, and the other group comprised people of similar ages who had no record of being in a car accident (as a driver, not a passenger) over the same 10-year span. (The researchers couldn't be sure that the accident was the driver's fault—there was no way to tell, based on the data. And determining blame in accidents is sometimes subjective.) *Then researchers analyzed who in the accident group had taken any of the following drugs within one month of the accident...*

Antipsychotics

Thorazine (*chlorpromazine*)	Zyprexa (*olanzapine*)
Depixol (*flupentixol*)	Seroquel (*quetiapine*)
Loxitane (*loxapine*)	Risperdal (*risperidone*)

Antidepressants

SSRIs (selective serotonin reuptake inhibitors)

Prozac (*fluoxetine*)	Celexa (*citalopram*)
Paxil (*paroxetine*)	Lexapro (*escitalopram*)

Zoloft (*sertraline*)

Tricyclic antidepressants:

Trofanil (*imipramine*)   Elavil (*amitriptyline*)

"Others":

Wellbutrin (*bupropion*)   Cymbalta (*duloxetine*)

Effexor (*venlafaxine*)

Benzodiazepines *Hypnotics*

Halcion (*triazolam*)   Dalame (*flurazepam*)

Anxiolytics:

Xanax (*alprazolam*)   Valium (*diazepam*)

Klonopin (*clonazepam*)   Ativan (lorazepam)

"Z-drugs" or sleeping pills

Ambien (*zolpidem*)   Sonata (*zaleplon*)

Then researchers compared people of the same age and gender in both groups to see whether those who had taken any of the drugs mentioned above were more likely to have been in car accidents.

Impaired Driving Skills

Only two categories of drugs—antipsychotic drugs and "other" antidepressants—were not associated with a higher risk of having a car accident while every other category was.

It is, of course, possible that the underlying medical conditions that caused people to take the drugs—depression, anxiety and insomnia—contributed to the car accidents. Future research will need to address that. But there is some evidence that the drugs themselves may have played a role.

Many psychotropic drugs impair cognitive and psychomotor abilities—and of course, cognitive and psychomotor abilities are crucial for driving. While on these drugs, you might feel more drowsy or more confused, and your reflexes might be slower. All of these things may negatively impact your judgment and coordination.

Researchers aren't exactly sure why antipsychotic drugs and "other" antidepressants weren't shown to be associated with car crashes. It could be due to the smaller number of subjects taking these drugs in the study…or it could be that people on these particular drugs drive less often…or it could be that these drugs impair cognitive and psychomotor abilities less than the other drugs mentioned above.

Protect Yourself on the Road

If you take any of the types of drugs listed above that were associated with having car accidents, here's some advice...

For those who take the medication in the morning, ask your doctor whether you can take it at night instead. The effects of many psychotropic drugs are strongest after you first take them, and since people tend to drive most in the daytime, this simple switch might help.

Ask your physician if you can take a lower dosage of the drug or possibly be weaned off the drug altogether. Perhaps you can use a natural treatment or make a lifestyle change instead.

If you have to stay on the drug and there is someone else who can drive you places (such as a spouse, sibling, child or friend), see if it's possible to become a passenger for at least the time being.

People who must drive: Stay extra alert while you're on the road, drive slowly and, of course, wear your seatbelt. And be sure not to drive if you are tired or upset.

CHAPTER 8

Medication Smarts

Five Medication Mistakes You Never Want to Make

Albert W. Wu, MD, MPH, an internist and a professor of medicine, surgery and health policy & management at The Johns Hopkins Bloomberg School of Public Health and the director of the Center for Health Services and Outcomes Research, both in Baltimore. He was a member of the committee formed by the Institute of Medicine to identify and prevent medication errors.

Chewing a pill when it is meant to be swallowed might taste pretty bad, but it wouldn't necessarily be dangerous, right? Wrong—it can be fatal if too much of the active ingredient is released at one time.

This is just one of the preventable medication errors that occur regularly in our country—in fact, at least 100,000 Americans are hospitalized from such mistakes every year. How could something as simple as taking a medication go so wrong?

Here's how some of the most common medication mistakes can occur—and how to avoid them…

MISTAKE #1: **Not verifying the instructions on e-prescriptions.** Prescription pads are quickly becoming a thing of the past. Instead, your doctor now may enter your prescription into a computer, which electronically transmits it to your pharmacy. The good news is e-prescriptions solve the problem of illegible handwriting and help stop errors. For example, if your doctor enters a dose of a drug that is too low or too high for any patient, the computer will flag it. In hospitals, computerized prescribing has reduced medication errors by up to 85%. But mistakes still happen.

How errors can occur: Let's say that your doctor wants you to take a long-acting diabetes medication only once a day, but the computer's default setting, which comes up automatically, calls for twice-daily dosing. If he/she does not notice, the computer will send that information to the pharmacy. The level of medication in your body could become too high, and blood sugar could drop dangerously low.

My advice: Always ask your doctor how to take medication—how much... how frequently...what time of day...and with or without food. Write all this information down. Then check this information on the drug label when you pick up the prescription. If there's any discrepancy between what the doctor told you and what the label says, the pharmacist should contact your doctor.

MISTAKE #2: Not discussing the name of the drug with the doctor. There are more than 10,000 prescription drugs and some 300,000 over-the-counter (OTC) medications. Many have similar-sounding—and similarly spelled—names that are easily confused.

How errors can occur: Your doctor might inadvertently key in clonazepam (an antianxiety drug) instead of clonidine (for high blood pressure).

My advice: Ask your doctor to pronounce and/or write down for you the name of the drug he is prescribing. Repeat the name to make sure you have it right. When you pick up the drug, say the name aloud to the pharmacist and/or show him the paper so you can double-check that you're getting the right medication.

MISTAKE #3: Accepting an "average" dose. When prescribing a drug, most doctors choose an average dose that would cover people of various sizes and ages. It's approximate, not precise.

How errors can occur: Suppose that you need a 10-mg dose of Lasix (a diuretic), based on your body weight, gender and age. If the lowest dose from the manufacturer is 20 mg, that's probably what you'll get (you could be instructed to cut the pill in half, but that may not happen). Too-high doses increase the risk for side effects and other complications.

My advice: Tell your doctor that you'd like to start low. Ask for the lowest possible effective dose. You and your doctor can increase it later.

MISTAKE #4: Splitting pills that should never be split. Some people split their pills in half to save money. But some pills can be safely split... others can't.

How errors can occur: Splitting a time-released medication could cause all of the active ingredient to be released at once. Or the pill's protective coating may be damaged, causing the drug to be broken down in the stomach rather than in the intestine, so it is not properly absorbed.

My advice: If cost is an issue, tell your doctor. There might be a lower-priced medication that will work as well. For example, a generic antiviral can cost $9, while a brand-name option could be as much as $65.

MISTAKE #5: **Taking double doses.** This happens a lot—mainly because people don't realize what the active ingredients are in the various drugs they're taking.

How errors can occur: Let's say that you take OTC acetaminophen for joint pain. But maybe you are taking a cold medicine that also contains acetaminophen. Then your doctor or dentist gives you a prescription for Tylenol with codeine (which contains even more acetaminophen). You could wind up getting a double or even triple dose.

Too much acetaminophen can cause liver damage, particularly when combined with alcohol.

My advice: Even though the active ingredients are listed on package inserts or packaging for all drugs, ask your pharmacist about this when you pick up a medication. If any active ingredients are found in more than one of the drugs you take, ask your pharmacist and/or doctor if the combined dosage is safe.

Vital Questions for Your Pharmacist

Do yourself a favor—the next time you pick up a prescription talk to your pharmacist. This is one of the best ways to avoid medication errors. *Key questions to ask your pharmacist…*

- **What is the active ingredient in this medicine?**
- **Should I avoid any other medicines, supplements, foods or drinks when taking this drug?***
- **Is there anything I should watch for**—such as allergic reactions or other side effects?
- **Should I take this medication on an empty stomach or with food?**
- **What should I do if I miss a dose…or use too much?**
- **Will I need any tests to check on the medicine's effectiveness**—such as blood tests?
- **How and where should I store this medicine?**

*You also can check for interactions at PDRhealth.com.

Are You Overdosing on OTC Drugs?

Suzy Cohen, RPh, a licensed pharmacist in Boulder, Colorado, and the author of the *"Dear Pharmacist"* syndicated column, which reaches 20 million readers nationwide, *The 24-Hour Pharmacist, Diabetes Without Drugs* and *Drug Muggers*. SuzyCohen.com

Painkillers, heartburn drugs and laxatives are among the worst offenders. We hear a lot about overuse of prescription drugs. That's because every year, more than 20,000 Americans die from a prescription drug overdose. About 75% of those fatalities are from painkillers such as *oxycodone* (OxyContin) and *hydrocodone* (Vicodin). But there's another unexpected threat—and that's overdosing on over-the-counter (OTC) painkillers.

Believe it or not, the main culprit is acetaminophen—the common pain reliever in Tylenol and other brands. It hospitalizes 30,000 people annually, many of whom develop acute liver failure.

Studies show that one-half to two-thirds of acetaminophen overdoses are the result of victims' poor understanding of the product's dosing instructions. One study published in the *Journal of General Internal Medicine* tested 500 people to determine their knowledge about and use of acetaminophen.

By their answers, many of the study participants showed that they would overdose—24% by using one product and unknowingly taking more than the safe limit of 4,000 mg (4 g) every 24 hours...and about 46% by using two acetaminophen-containing products at the same time without realizing the combined dosage would be an overdose.

The same misuse of medications and misunderstanding of labels occurs with other types of OTC medications described throughout this article—with potentially disastrous long-term consequences for health. *Here's how to make sure that you don't overdose on or overuse OTC drugs...*

Acetaminophen

Acetaminophen is the most commonly used OTC drug in the US—every week, one out of every five adults takes it. And for good reason—the drug works fast to reduce pain and fever. In fact, acetaminophen works so well, it's the main pain-relieving, fever-lowering ingredient in many OTC products for headache, arthritis, back pain, colds, coughs, sinus problems and more. But the effectiveness and availability of the ingredient is a setup for overdosing.

Fortunately, a few simple precautions can help prevent an acetaminophen overdose...

•**Read the labels and do the math.** Read the ingredient list on every OTC drug you take and know which contain acetaminophen and how much. Keep careful track of your daily intake—and don't ever take more than 1,000 mg at any one time or exceed 4,000 mg in a day. The more acetaminophen-containing products you take, the more likely it is you'll overdose.

Example: In the *Journal of General Internal Medicine* overdose study, three drug combinations were most likely to cause an overdose—a pain reliever and a PM pain reliever…a pain reliever and a cough and cold medicine…a sinus medication and a PM pain reliever.

•**Know if you are at high risk—and be extra-cautious if you are.** In the overdose study, people who were "heavy users" of acetaminophen (taking it a couple of days a week or more) were more likely to underestimate their intake—and to overdose.

Important: If you suffer from chronic pain, see your primary care physician or a pain specialist, and ask for a stronger medication that is taken once or twice a day. That way, you won't have to take as many OTC painkillers.

•**Know the signs of an overdose.** An overdose of acetaminophen typically causes nausea and vomiting, sweating, yellowing of the skin and eyes and a general feeling of flulike illness. Within one to three days, it causes pain in the upper right quadrant of the abdomen (the location of the liver). If you develop those symptoms after regular use of acetaminophen (or after a single dose that is excessive)—seek immediate medical care.

Self-defense: Call 911 or go to a hospital emergency department if you have severe symptoms, such as gasping for air. The standard treatment for acetaminophen overdose is n-acetyl-cysteine (NAC), an antioxidant that reverses liver toxicity, often given intravenously. Although NAC capsules are available at health-food stores, it's best to be treated by medical personnel since an overdose is a serious medical condition. If you suspect that you may be experiencing symptoms of an overdose, you can call a 24-hour poison control center such as the National Capital Poison Center at 800-222-1222.

Proton Pump Inhibitors (PPIs)

These popular drugs work by slowing down your body's production of stomach acid, preventing and relieving the symptoms of heartburn. They also are used to treat indigestion (dyspepsia), ulcers and other upper gastrointestinal (GI) problems. Two kinds are available OTC—*lansoprazole* (Prevacid 24HR) and *omeprazole* (Prilosec OTC, Zegerid OTC).

The danger: These drugs, if taken daily, should not be used for more than two weeks without a doctor's approval, according to label instructions. Studies show that overuse can increase risk for hip, wrist or spine fractures in adults over age 50...and cardiac arrhythmias, intense diarrhea, colds, flu and pneumonia, and vitamin and mineral deficiencies in users of all ages. In addition, when you stop taking one of these drugs abruptly, it can trigger rebound acid hypersecretion—a surge of stomach acid that worsens symptoms, forcing you back on the drug for relief.

Self-defense: Slowly wean yourself off long-term use of a PPI. Speak to your doctor about the best way to do this. Afterward, treat heartburn with OTC antacids, a much safer choice (follow label instructions).

Nasal Decongestants

Many people suffer from rhinitis medicamentosa (RM)—a chronically stuffy nose caused by overuse of nasal decongestant spray. For example, you might use a spray, such as Afrin or Neo-Synephrine containing the ingredient *oxymetazoline* or *phenylephrine*, during a cold or allergy season. It provides relief, but there is "rebound congestion" when the spray wears off. You use it again... there is rebound congestion...and you use it again. Soon, you have RM—and are addicted to the nasal spray for "relief."

Self-defense: If you are addicted to a nasal spray, wean yourself off slowly. (*Examples*: Alternate nostrils with each use, rather than spraying both nostrils. Or use the spray only at bedtime to get you through the night.) As you decrease use, try a nonmedicated saline spray or a menthol nasal spray and a humidifier or steam vaporizer. You might also ask your doctor for a short-term prescription for nasal corticosteroids, which will relieve congestion while you withdraw from the spray. Plus, address underlying health problems that may cause nasal congestion, such as food allergies or structural problems in the sinuses.

Laxatives

Constipation is a common problem, and daily use of OTC laxatives, such as Miralax and Milk of Magnesia, is frequently the "solution."

The danger: Laxative overuse can lead to abdominal cramping, nausea and vomiting, blood in the stool, mineral deficiencies, electrolyte imbalances that cause heart and kidney damage—and, in rare cases, death.

Self-defense: Wean yourself slowly off laxatives. For example, start by switching from daily use to every-other-day use.

As you're reducing use, add more fiber to your diet, with fruits, vegetables, whole grains and beans—and, if necessary, take a daily fiber supplement—to help ensure regular bowel movements. Take a probiotic, a supplement of "friendly" bacteria that aids digestive health. Other digestive aids that can help cure constipation include aloe vera, essential fatty acids and digestive enzymes. Talk to your doctor about which of these digestive aids might work best for you. Drink water throughout the day and exercise regularly, which stimulates bowels.

Stay Safe

Keep all your prescriptions at the same pharmacy. That way, your pharmacist has your complete medication profile and can accurately advise you about your OTC medications.

When buying an OTC product, ask your pharmacist to check for interactions between your prescription drugs and your OTC choices. You are not being a "pest"—the pharmacist wants to help keep you safe.

Prescription Drugs That Make You Sick

Armon B. Neel, Jr., PharmD, a certified geriatric pharmacist and coauthor of *Are Your Prescriptions Killing You? How to Prevent Dangerous Interactions, Avoid Deadly Side Effects, and Be Healthier with Fewer Drugs.* MedicationXpert.com

When your doctor pulls out his/her prescription pad, you probably assume that your health problem will soon be improving. Sure, there may be a side effect or two—perhaps an occasional upset stomach or a mild headache. But overall you will be better off, right?

Not necessarily. While it's true that many drugs can help relieve symptoms and sometimes even cure certain medical conditions, a number of popular medications actually cause disease—not simply side effects—while treating the original problem.

Here's what happens: Your kidney and liver are the main organs that break down drugs and eliminate them from your body. But these organs weaken as you age. Starting as early as your 20s and 30s, you lose 1% of liver and kidney function every year. As a result, drugs can build up in your body (particularly if you take more than one), become toxic, damage crucial organs such as the heart and brain—and trigger disease.

Older adults are at greatest risk for this problem because the body becomes increasingly less efficient at metabolizing drugs with age. But no one is exempt from the risk. *To protect yourself—or a loved one...*

Dementia

Many drugs can cause symptoms, such as short-term memory loss, confusion and agitation, that patients (and physicians) frequently mistake for dementia. The main offenders are anticholinergic medications, which treat a variety of conditions by blocking the activity of the neurotransmitter acetylcholine.

Hundreds of medications are anticholinergic, and it's likely that any class of drugs beginning with anti- is in this category—for example, antihistamines and antispasmodics. Cholesterol-lowering statins also can cause dementia-like symptoms.

Other offenders: Beta-blockers (for high blood pressure or cardiac arrhythmias)...benzodiazepines (for anxiety)...narcotics...tricyclic antidepressants...anticonvulsants...muscle relaxants...sleeping pills...fluoroquinolone antibiotics...heartburn drugs (H2 receptor antagonists and proton-pump inhibitors)...antipsychotics...nitrates (for heart disease)...and sulfonylurea derivatives (for diabetes).

My advice: If you or a loved one has been diagnosed with dementia, the patient should immediately undergo a comprehensive medication review— drug-induced dementia usually can be reversed by stopping the offending drug (or drugs). A competent physician or consultant pharmacist can always find an alternative drug to use.

Surprising threat: Even general anesthesia can cause weeks or months of dementia-like confusion (and an incorrect diagnosis of Alzheimer's) in an older person as the drug slowly leaves the body.

The anesthesia is collected in the fat cells in the body, and normal cognition may take months to return. The longer a person is under anesthesia, the longer it takes to recover.

Cancer

Medications known as biologics are frequently used to treat autoimmune diseases such as inflammatory bowel disease, or IBD (including Crohn's disease and ulcerative colitis) and rheumatoid arthritis.

This class of drugs includes *adalimumab* (Humira), *certolizumab* (Cimzia), *etanercept* (Enbrel), *golimumab* (Simponi) and *infliximab* (Remicade).

Important finding: The use of biologics was linked to more than triple the risk for lymphoma, breast, pancreatic and other cancers in a study that was published in *The Journal of the American Medical Association.*

The danger: While these medications may have a role in the treatment of autoimmune diseases, they often are carelessly prescribed by primary care physicians. For example, a biologic that is intended for IBD may be mistakenly prescribed for irritable bowel syndrome (IBS), a far less serious digestive disorder.

If you are prescribed a biologic for IBD: Before starting the drug, ask for a comprehensive workup to confirm the diagnosis. This may include lab tests, imaging tests (ultrasound, CT or MRI), a biopsy and a stool analysis (to rule out C. difficile and other bowel infections that would require an antibiotic). Do not take a biologic for IBS.

If you are prescribed a biologic for rheumatoid arthritis: Before starting the medication, ask your doctor for a comprehensive workup to confirm the diagnosis, including lab tests and imaging tests (X-ray, ultrasound or MRI). Do not take a biologic for osteoarthritis. Besides increasing cancer risk, the suppression of the immune system opens the door for serious bacterial and viral infections.

Diabetes

Many commonly prescribed drugs increase risk for type 2 diabetes. These medications include statins…beta-blockers…antidepressants…antipsychotics…steroids…and alpha-blockers prescribed for prostate problems and high blood pressure.

Safer alternatives to discuss with your doctor, consultant pharmacist or other health-care professional…

If you're prescribed a beta-blocker: Ask about using a calcium-channel blocker instead. *Diltiazem* (Tiazac) has the fewest side effects. The 24-hour sustained-release dose provides the best control.

If you're prescribed an antidepressant: Ask about *venlafaxine* (Effexor), a selective serotonin and norepinephrine reuptake inhibitor (SSNRI) antidepressant that treats depression and anxiety and has been shown to cause fewer problems for diabetic patients than any of the older selective serotonin reuptake inhibitor (SSRI) drugs.

If you're prescribed an alpha-blocker: For prostate problems, rather than taking the alpha-blocker *tamsulosin* (Flomax), ask about using *dutasteride*

(Avodart) or *finasteride* (Proscar). For high blood pressure, ask about a calcium-channel blocker drug.

Heart Disease

Nonsteroidal anti-inflammatory drugs (NSAIDs), frequently taken to ease pain due to arthritis, other joint problems or headaches, are widely known to damage the digestive tract. What's less well known is that NSAIDs have been found to increase the risk for cardiovascular disease.

My advice: No one over the age of 50 with mild-to-moderate pain should use an NSAID.

Fortunately, there is an excellent alternative. A daily dose of 50 mg of the prescription non-narcotic pain reliever *tramadol* (Ultracet, Ultram) and/or 325 mg of *acetaminophen* (Tylenol) works well and has less risk for adverse effects. Acetaminophen, taken in appropriate doses (less than 3,000 mg daily) without alcohol use, is safe and effective. I also recommend 3 g to 4 g of fish oil daily—it has been shown to effectively treat joint pain. Talk to your doctor first because fish oil may increase risk for bleeding.

The Very Best Drug Self-Defense

If you're over age 60—especially if you take more than one medication or suffer drug side effects—it's a good idea to ask your physician to work with a consulting pharmacist who is skilled in medication management. A consulting pharmacist has been trained in drug-therapy management and will work with your physician to develop a drug-management plan that will avoid harmful drugs. These services are relatively new and may not be covered by insurance, so be sure to check with your provider.

To find a consulting pharmacist in your area, go to the website of the American Society of Consultant Pharmacists, ASCPcom, and click on SENIORX.

Also helpful: Make sure that a drug you've been prescribed does not appear on the "Beers Criteria for Potentially Inappropriate Medication Use in Older Adults." Originally developed by Mark Beers, editor of *The Merck Manual of Medical Information*, the list has been recently updated by The American Geriatrics Society. To download the list for free, go to AmericanGeriatrics.org and search "Beers criteria."

Popular Drugs That Have Surprising Side Effects

Robert Steven Gold, RPh, a hospital pharmacist and affiliate instructor of clinical pharmacy at Purdue University in West Lafayette, Indiana. He is the author of *Are Your Meds Making You Sick? A Pharmacist's Guide to Avoiding Dangerous Drug Interactions, Reactions and Side Effects.*

Medication is given to patients to help them, not harm them, which is why it is so hard to comprehend that the side effects and interactions from medications cause more deaths annually than homicides, car accidents and airplane crashes combined. This means that, every year, approximately 100,000 deaths in the US are caused, in part, by dangerous drug reactions.

Some medication side effects are easy to recognize, such as an upset stomach after taking aspirin or confusion from sedatives. Other side effects—as well as drug interactions—may be unexpected and harder to recognize.

For example…

Irregular Heartbeat

Culprit: Levofloxacin (Levaquin), a broad-spectrum antibiotic given for infections. The fluoroquinolone class of antibiotics, which includes *levofloxacin* and *ciprofloxacin* (Cipro), has been linked to torsades de pointes, a rare but dangerous heart irregularity (arrhythmia) that can cause instant death in some cases.

Warning: Patients who take one of these antibiotics along with a thiazide diuretic, such as *hydrochlorothiazide* (Microzide), may have a higher risk for heart irregularities.

New development: A study published in *The New England Journal of Medicine* has found that *azithromycin* (Zithromax and others), an antibiotic used to treat bacterial infections, may increase risk for irregular heartbeat and sudden death in patients with, or at risk for, heart disease.

Solution: If you take any of these antibiotics and experience a change in your heart's rhythm (a feeling of fluttering in the heart or a heart rate greater than 100 beats per minute), go to the emergency room. Episodes that last for more than about 10 seconds can cause a loss of consciousness and sometimes seizures.

Burning Rash on Upper Body

Culprit: Sulfamethoxazole-trimethoprim (Bactrim), a sulfonamide antibiotic, used to treat intestinal and urinary tract infections and pneumonia. This class of antibiotics can lead to Stevens-Johnson syndrome (SJS), an immune reaction that causes flulike symptoms, including fever, followed by a painful, itchy rash that spreads, blisters and can become infected. Sores in the mouth and mucous membranes also are common.

SJS is rare, affecting one to three patients per 100,000, but it can be life-threatening. About 25% to 35% of patients who have an extensive rash (covering 30% or more of the body) die from it.

Solution: If you take sulfamethoxazole and trimethoprim or another sulfonamide antibiotic and experience any of the side effects described earlier, go to the emergency room. Patients with SJS are hospitalized and given the same treatments as burn victims.

Unexplained Bruises

Culprit: Warfarin (Coumadin), a "blood thinner" that inhibits blood clotting and often is prescribed to patients with heart disease or who have had a heart attack. Warfarin, as well as other anticlotting drugs, can make the blood so thin that bleeding occurs from the stomach, intestine or gums. And since bleeding can take longer to stop, blood can leak from a capillary and cause a bruise without an injury.

An article by Canadian researchers published in *Annals of Internal Medicine* analyzing the results of 33 previous studies, found that patients taking warfarin had about a one in 39 chance of serious bleeding. About one in eight patients with major bleeding episodes died.

Solution: Warfarin can be a life-saving drug if you need it, but you should work closely with your doctor to find the dosage that is best for you. Also, it's crucial to be aware that other medications, supplements and even foods can thin your blood. These medications include nonsteroidal anti-inflammatory drugs (NSAIDs), such as aspirin and *ibuprofen* (Motrin), and *clopidogrel* (Plavix), an antiplatelet drug—all of which have bleeding as a side effect. Before taking any other drug, let your doctor know that you're also taking warfarin.

Caution: Many herbs and supplements, such as fish oil, licorice, ginseng and coenzyme Q10, can increase/worsen the effects of warfarin.

Also important: Foods that are high in vitamin K, such as spinach and kale, affect the rate at which your blood clots and could require a change in your dose of warfarin. If you take a blood thinner, speak to your doctor about the effects of other medications, supplements and foods on your blood.

Stomach or Esophagus Ulcers

Culprit: Alendronate (Fosamax), taken to prevent/treat osteoporosis. Alendronate is known to cause stomach ulcers in about 1% of patients and ulcers in the esophagus in up to 2%. These are small percentages, but the risk rises when patients also take an NSAID, such as ibuprofen or *naproxen* (Aleve).

Solution: If you need a drug such as alendronate to preserve bone strength, changing how you take the medication can reduce the side effects.

Examples: Take alendronate first thing in the morning when your stomach is empty, washing it down with six to eight ounces of plain water. Taking it with some beverages or foods, particularly orange juice or acidic foods, increases the risk for ulcers. Don't lie down for 30 minutes after taking it—this can cause stomach acids to reach, and damage, the esophagus.

Also important: Avoid NSAIDs. Take *acetaminophe*n (Tylenol), a non-NSAID painkiller.

Persistent Muscle Pain

Culprit: Gemfibrozil (Lopid), a fibrate medication that's used to reduce triglycerides and increase HDL "good" cholesterol, taken with a statin drug.

Doctors routinely tell patients that cholesterol-lowering statins, such as *atorvastatin* (Lipitor) or *simvastatin* (Zocor), may cause muscle pain. But they often neglect to mention that other cholesterol medications can have the same effect. Up to 30% of patients who take a statin experience some degree of muscle pain. The risk is higher when patients also take gemfibrozil or another fibrate drug because this medication decreases levels of liver enzymes that are needed to break down statins.

Result: Statin levels gradually rise in the body, which increases the risk for muscle pain.

Solution: If you're taking both a fibrate and a statin, ask your doctor if the statin dose is low enough to prevent side effects.

Tremors

Culprit: Metoclopramide (Reglan), a medication for heartburn, plus *prochlorperazine*, a medication to relieve nausea.

Metoclopramide causes Tardive dyskinesia (uncontrolled muscle movements, especially in the face) in about 20% of patients who take it for three months or longer. It blocks the effects of dopamine, a brain chemical that plays a role in cognition and movement, the loss of which also occurs in Parkinson's patients. Prochlorperazine also blocks the effects of dopamine. When these drugs are taken together, the risk for movement disorders is much higher.

Solution: Switch to a different heartburn drug—for example, an antacid or a medication such as *cimetidine* (Tagamet), an H2 blocker, that does not typically block dopamine.

Important: Tremors caused by medication may not appear for up to six months. If you are experiencing any kind of movement disorder, ask your doctor to review all of your medications, not just the ones that you've recently started.

Steps to Protect Yourself

Speak to each of your physicians about all the medications you are taking. Alert your prescribing doctor if you experience any side effects when starting a new drug. Doctors often can find an effective substitute.

Very important: It's best to always use the same pharmacy or pharmacy chain. Every medication that you take, or have taken, is stored in the pharmacy's computer, which identifies potential drug interactions. Ask the pharmacist to look up your record when you are picking up a prescription.

Medications That Hurt Your Eyes

Jeffrey R. Anshel, OD, optometrist and founder of Corporate Vision Consulting, which addresses visual demands in the workplace. He has written six books on computer vision concerns and nutritional influences on vision, the latest being The *Ocular Nutrition Handbook.*

Are your eyes dry or sensitive to light? Do you have blurred vision or "floaters"? These and other eye problems could be side effects of common medications.

Few people make the connection between changes in their eyes and medications they take—yet the truth is that many prescription and over-the-counter drugs cause ocular side effects. *Here are common symptoms and the drugs that could be causing them...*

Important: Contact your physician (eye doctor or primary care) if you have any of these symptoms. Most are not dangerous, and minor eye problems may be a reasonable trade-off for a potentially lifesaving drug. Always bring with you to the doctor a complete list of the medications you take—prescription and over-the-counter—and the doses. Stopping the medications can reverse the symptoms in many cases.

•**Abnormalities in pupil size.** Discrepancies in how your pupils react to light (called aniscoria) can be caused by a variety of medications, including Catapres (for hypertension), Donnatal (irritable bowel syndrome/ulcers), Humulin (diabetes) and Tavist (allergies).

If your pupils aren't always the same size—especially if only one pupil is abnormally enlarged—it's important to go to the emergency room immediately. The brain controls pupil size, so a disturbance there can cause pupils to be different sizes.

•**Cataracts.** If you live long enough, you eventually will develop cataracts (lenses that have clouded over, making it more difficult to see). Certain drugs may speed the process, including Coumadin (for heart disease), Plaquenil (malaria, rheumatoid arthritis and lupus) and most steroids.

•**Difficulty focusing.** The medical term for this condition is "accommodative insufficiency." It grows more common with age and also is a side effect of some medications. These include Adipex (for obesity), *methyclothiazide* (hypertension), Norpramin (depression) and Xanax (anxiety).

•**Double or blurred vision.** There are many potential causes for seeing double or for vision that suddenly blurs. Medications that can cause this include Adipex (for obesity), Celebrex (inflammation), Lamictal (seizures), *lovastatin* (elevated cholesterol), Tylenol (pain relief) and Zantac (ulcers).

If your blurred or double vision is sudden, severe and unrelenting, go to the emergency room immediately. This visual impairment is not only unsafe (for instance, when you are driving), but it could be a sign of a serious medical problem such as a stroke or brain lesion.

•**Dry eyes.** Many factors (including computer use, wearing contact lenses and allergies) can reduce tear production and cause dry eyes—and so can certain medications, such as Actifed (for allergies), Catapres (hypertension), Detrol (bladder control) and Paxil (depression).

Until you see your doctor, self-treatment options for dry eyes include blinking as often as possible...use of artificial tear solutions (available in drugstores and chain stores)...avoiding irritants, including eye makeup and air pollution...and wearing sunglasses. Or try an oral gamma-linolenic acid (GLA) product such as BioTears.

•**Eye irritation.** Redness in the whites of your eyes or irritations on your eyelids can be caused by medications such as Aricept (taken to improve cognitive loss), Cardizem (heart disease), *methyclothiazide* (heart disease) and Voltaren (rheumatoid arthritis, osteoporosis).

•**Floaters and other visual disturbances.** Flashes of light or color, floaters and other visual disturbances can occur for a host of reasons, including as a side effect of a drug. Medications linked to visual disturbances include Benadryl (for allergies), Cardizem (heart disease), and Xanax (anxiety).

The causes of visual disturbances can range from inconsequential to potentially serious, so they should be checked out by your eye doctor as quickly as possible. This is especially true if you suddenly see flashes of light or if numerous new floaters appear—that could be a sign of a retinal detachment.

•**Light sensitivity.** Though there are other possible causes, light sensitivity may be a side effect of drugs (including recreational drugs such as cocaine and amphetamines). Drugs linked with light sensitivity include Diabinese (for diabetes), Dilantin (epilepsy), Lipitor (high cholesterol/heart disease), Pepcid (gastric ulcers) and Viagra (erectile dysfunction). If light sensitivity is severe and your pupils are enlarged—especially if only one pupil is enlarged—go to the ER. It could be a sign of stroke or a brain tumor.

•**Yellowed eyes.** Several conditions can cause the white parts of the eye to turn yellow, including illness, sun exposure and drugs such as Diabinese (for diabetes) and Librium (anxiety). Yellowing may be a sign of cirrhosis or hepatitis. It is important to see your doctor quickly to have this checked out.

Drugs That Work Against Each Other

David Lee, PharmD, PhD, assistant professor in the College of Pharmacy at Oregon State University in Portland. Dr. Lee is also a coauthor of a recent paper on therapeutic competition that was published in the journal *PLOS ONE*.

Cynthia Kuhn, PhD, professor in the department of pharmacology at Duke University School of Medicine, Durham, North Carolina, and codirector of Brainworks, a Duke program that develops education programs about the brain. She is a coauthor of *Buzzed: The Straight Facts About the Most Used and Abused Drugs from Alcohol to Ecstasy.*

Most people who have a chronic health problem such as osteoarthritis, high blood pressure or diabetes are accustomed to taking medication to help control their symptoms.

But if you have more than one chronic condition—and take medication for each of them—you could be setting yourself up for other problems.

The risk that often goes undetected: Taking medication prescribed for one disease may actually worsen another health problem. This situation, known as "therapeutic competition," has received surprisingly little attention from the medical profession.

According to the federal Substance Abuse and Mental Health Services Administration, emergency room visits involving adverse reactions to pharmaceuticals increased 82.9% between 2005 and 2009 (from 1.2 million to over 2.2 million), particularly among patients 65 and older.

Caution: The risk for drug interactions is highest among the elderly. They tend to use the most drugs, and their bodies metabolize (break down) drugs more slowly than younger adults.

How Interactions Happen

Patients who use medications appropriately—taking the prescribed doses for only particular conditions and regularly reviewing drug use with a physician—are unlikely to have serious problems.

Main risks: Different drugs prescribed by more than one doctor…using drugs to treat conditions for which they weren't originally prescribed (many people stockpile leftover drugs and use them later, possibly for unrelated conditions)…or using a drug that was appropriate initially but might be dangerous when combined with drugs a patient has subsequently started taking.

Protect yourself by frequently updating a list of the drugs and supplements you take. Review the list with every doctor at every office visit and whenever a new drug is prescribed.

Are You At Risk?

Therapeutic competition can occur at any time in a person's life. But the risk increases with age—the older we get, the more likely we are to have chronic medical conditions and use more medications. Because our bodies metabolize medication less efficiently as we age, we're also more likely to develop side effects that can worsen other health problems.

Modern medicine has not done very much to help the situation. For one thing, polypharmacy—the use of multiple medications—has become more common than ever before.

For people with more than one chronic medical condition, frequent conflicts occur if you have...

•**High Blood Pressure.** If you also have chronic obstructive pulmonary disease (COPD), drugs that you take to ease your breathing, such as the beta-adrenergic agonist *albuterol* (Proventil) or a corticosteroid, may raise your blood pressure.

If you are also being treated for depression, an antidepressant such as *venlafaxine* (Effexor) or *duloxetine* (Cymbalta) could push your blood pressure higher. COX-2 inhibitors such as *celecoxib* (Celebrex), commonly used for osteoarthritis, also may increase blood pressure.

•**Diabetes.** Corticosteroids taken for COPD can raise blood sugar levels, worsening diabetes. If you have an enlarged prostate and take an alpha-blocker such as *tamsulosin* (Flomax) or a beta-blocker such as *atenolol* (Tenormin) for high blood pressure, the drug can mask symptoms of low blood sugar, such as shakiness.

•**COPD.** If you also have high blood pressure or angina and take a nonselective beta-blocker such as propranolol (Inderal), the drug could worsen lung symptoms.

•**Heart Disease.** COPD drugs, including albuterol...tricyclic antidepressants such as *imipramine* (Tofranil), taken for depression...and COX-2 inhibitors for osteoarthritis also can make heart disease worse.

•**Atrial Fibrillation.** Osteoporosis drugs, including bisphosphonates such as *alendronate* (Fosamax)...and Alzheimer's drugs, including cholinesterase inhibitors such as *donepezil* (Aricept), may worsen atrial fibrillation.

•**Osteoporosis.** Corticosteroids used to treat COPD often lead to significant bone loss. Glitazones taken for diabetes and proton pump inhibitors such as *omeprazole* (Prilosec), commonly prescribed for gastroesophageal reflux disease (GERD), can accelerate bone loss.

•**Gerd or Peptic Ulcers.** *Warfarin* (Coumadin) or *clopidogrel* (Plavix), often prescribed for atrial fibrillation or heart disease, as well as nonsteroidal anti-inflammatory drugs (NSAIDs), can cause bleeding that worsens GERD and ulcers. Bisphosphonates taken for osteoporosis may aggravate esophageal damage that commonly occurs with GERD and ulcers.

Opioid Painkillers/Sedatives

Opioid painkillers, such as *hydrocodone* and *oxycodone*, have powerful effects on the central nervous system. Even on their own, they can suppress breathing when taken in high enough doses. The risk is much higher when they're combined with sedating drugs, such as those used to treat anxiety or insomnia. These include the benzodiazepine class of medications, such as *diazepam* (Valium) and *alprazolam* (Xanax).

Many people take these drugs in combination. For example, someone might take alprazolam for chronic anxiety, then add hydrocodone following an injury. The drugs often are prescribed by different doctors who don't know the patient's drug history.

What to do: Never combine prescription painkillers and sedatives without your doctor's okay.

Warfarin/Antibiotics/NSAIDs

The blood thinner *warfarin* (Coumadin) is notorious for interacting with other drugs. It has a narrow "therapeutic index," the difference between a helpful and a toxic dose. Drugs that increase the effects of warfarin can lead to uncontrolled bleeding.

Many antibiotics and antifungal drugs, including erythromycin, ciprofloxacin and ketoconazole, are broken down by the same liver enzyme that metabolizes warfarin. Taking warfarin and any of these drugs together may deplete the enzyme, leading to higher levels of warfarin in the body.

What to do: If you have an infection, your doctor can prescribe an antibiotic that is less likely to interact with warfarin. Antibiotics that are less likely to cause an interaction include penicillin, amoxicillin, ampicillin and tetracycline.

Caution: Warfarin may cause gastrointestinal bleeding when combined with aspirin, ibuprofen or other nonsteroidal anti-inflammatory drugs (NSAIDs). If you take warfarin and need a painkiller, *acetaminophen* (Tylenol) might be a better choice.

Multiple Antidepressants

Patients who combine selective serotonin reuptake inhibitor (SSRI) antidepressants, such as *fluoxetine* (Prozac) and *sertraline* (Zoloft), or who combine an SSRI with another type of antidepressant may experience serotonin syndrome, a rare but potentially fatal reaction.

Many antidepressants increase brain levels of serotonin, a chemical produced by some neurons (nerve cells). Patients who combine antidepressants or take too much of one can accumulate toxic levels of serotonin. This can cause dangerously elevated blood pressure, known as a hypertensive crisis.

Serotonin syndrome usually occurs when patients switch from an SSRI antidepressant to a monoamine oxidase inhibitor (MAOI), an older type of antidepressant, without allowing time for the first drug to wash out of the body.

What to do: Follow your doctor's instructions exactly when discontinuing an antidepressant. Most of these drugs have to be tapered—slowly decreasing the dose over a period of weeks—before starting a new drug.

Viagra/Nitrates

Men who take nitrate drugs (such as nitroglycerine) for heart problems should never take *sildenafil* (Viagra) without a doctor's supervision.

Viagra and similar drugs for treating erectile dysfunction cause blood vessels to relax. Nitrate drugs do the same thing. Combining them can cause a dangerous drop in blood pressure.

What to do: Men who take nitrates for heart problems can talk to their doctors about safer alternatives for treating erectile dysfunction, including vacuum devices or penile injections.

Acetaminophen from Multiple Products

Taken in excessive doses, the pain reliever *acetaminophen* (Tylenol) can cause liver damage.

Main risk: Combining acetaminophen—for treating arthritis pain, for example—with unrelated products (such as cold/flu remedies) that also contain acetaminophen.

What to do: When using acetaminophen, don't exceed the dose listed on the product label—and check labels to ensure that you don't take another product that contains acetaminophen simultaneously.

How to Protect Yourself

If you have more than one chronic condition and take two or more medications to treat them, it is crucial that you watch for signs of therapeutic competition, such as new symptoms that are unexplained or begin soon after a new medication is started. Any new health condition actually may be an adverse effect of medication.

Important steps to avoid therapeutic competition...

•**Try to cut back on the drugs you take.** The less medication you're on, the less likely one of your drugs will adversely affect another condition. Ask your doctor whether it's advisable to reduce the overall number of prescriptions you take. A drug you have been taking for years may no longer be necessary. You may also be able to make lifestyle changes—such as getting more exercise—that will allow you to cut back on blood pressure or diabetes medication.

•**Get the right medication.** If it seems that a drug is worsening another condition, ask your doctor about less harmful alternatives. Some medications are more selective—that is, their effects on the body are more focused on the target illness, making unintended consequences for other conditions less of a danger.

Example: Nonselective beta-blockers, such as propranolol, often worsen COPD symptoms, but medications with more selective action, such as *metoprolol* (Lopressor), are usually just as effective for the heart problem they're prescribed for without adversely affecting your lungs.

Get a Yearly Medication Check

If you suffer from multiple ailments, you need to tell all your doctors about the medications you take. Also, talk to your pharmacist each time you pick up a new prescription to make sure your drugs aren't working against each other.

To ensure that no drug-related problems develop: Once a year, have a pharmacist (ask one at your drugstore) review all your medications. This service includes a discussion of side effects, interactions and alternatives. For many people, Medicare Part D and some private health plans will pay for this service. If not, it usually costs less than $100.

Drugs Plus Supplements: Proceed with Caution

Leo Galland, MD, internist and director, Foundation for Integrated Medicine, New York City. Dr. Galland publishes a free newsletter, which includes more information about supplements and drugs. MDHeal.org

About 40% of Americans now take dietary supplements in the form of a vitamin, mineral, herb or other substance—and those 50 and older are more likely than younger folks to use supplements and, as a group, to take more medications. The sicker and more fragile you are, the greater the impact of an interaction. But in truth, anyone combining drugs and supplements is at risk for interactions—and the more drugs and supplements that you take, the greater the danger.

Surprisingly Common Interactions

Here are some of the more common medications people take and what supplements might cause dangerous interactions...

•**Blood-thinning drugs.** If you take *warfarin* or another blood-thinning drug (including aspirin), don't take ginkgo biloba, and ask your doctor about the advisability of taking vitamin E, since even the amount in a multivitamin can increase your risk for hemorrhage.

Two others to beware of: Ginseng and St. John's wort also can be dangerous for those on blood-thinning drugs, as they may prevent warfarin from working properly and increase risk for blood clots.

•**Statins.** If you take a statin drug, don't take vitamin E or St. John's wort because they may reduce the drug's effectiveness and leave you vulnerable to heart attack. It's well known that grapefruit can increase blood levels of some statin drugs to dangerously high levels, increasing the risk for liver or muscle damage, but you may not know that pomegranate and pomegranate extract can have the same effect.

•**Diuretics.** Anyone who takes a thiazide drug (such as *hydrochlorthiazide*) on its own or in combination with another blood pressure medication (such as an ACE inhibitor) should avoid the supplements white willow bark and ginkgo biloba—these can prevent the drugs from working properly, so patients may end up with elevated blood pressure. Horsetail, senna, cascara, licorice and uva ursi (all typically taken for bloating and water retention) boost the diuretic effect of thiazide drugs and can lead to dehydration and potassium depletion.

•**Antihypertensives.** People on ACE inhibitors for blood pressure, a category that includes *captopril* and *lisinopril* (Zestril and Prinivil), should avoid taking iron supplements within two hours of taking the medication because iron can interfere with absorption of the drug. Iron naturally present in food does not have the same effect. Also problematic is the supplement cayenne (sometimes referred to as capsicum or capsaicin), used as a digestive aid or for control of inflammation, which increases the side effects of ACE inhibitors, especially cough.

•**Oral diabetes medications.** If you are taking diabetes medicines such as *metformin* (Glucophage) or *glyburide* (Glynase), avoid ginkgo biloba because it can interfere with the effects of insulin and raise your blood sugar. Also use caution with the supplements vanadium, gymnema, chromium, ginseng and bitter melon, as these can dangerously depress blood sugar levels in sensitive individuals.

•**Antiarrhythmia drugs.** Patients who take the antiarrhythmia drug *digoxin* should never take supplemental forms of licorice (often used for cough or sore throat) because it can bring on severe—even fatal—arrhythmia. Others to avoid include pectin, a stool-bulking agent, because it reduces absorption of the digoxin, and ginseng, which binds with the digoxin, making it unavailable. Also avoid horsetail, senna and cascara, which can bring about dangerous reductions of potassium levels, which increase the risk for digoxin toxicity.

•**Antibiotics.** If you are on tetracycline or the antibiotic class known as quinolone antibiotics, which includes Cipro and *levofloxacin* (Levaquin), do not take minerals or eat mineral-rich foods within two hours of taking the drug—minerals such as calcium, magnesium, iron and zinc bind to these drugs and prevent their absorption. Dairy products and calcium-fortified juices should also be avoided within two hours of antibiotics because the calcium can block drug absorption.

•**Thyroid medications.** If you take a thyroid medication such as *levothyroxine* (Synthroid), do not take any iron, calcium or aluminum (found in antacids) within four hours because they interfere with absorption of the drug.

Ask an Expert

Supplements should be used with the same care as drugs. It's best to take them under the supervision of a doctor (such as a naturopath) who is specially trained in their use or to ask your pharmacist for advice.

When Drugs and Juices Don't Mix

Beverly J. McCabe-Sellers, PhD, RD, former professor of dietetics and nutrition at the University of Arkansas for Medical Sciences in Little Rock for more than 20 years and coeditor of the *Handbook of Food-Drug Interactions*.

I f you take any kind of prescription or over-the-counter (OTC) medication, you may be unwittingly reducing its benefits and/or increasing its risks by drinking certain beverages when you swallow the drug. The potentially harmful interactions also may occur if you drink the beverage hours before or after taking the medication. *For example…*

Dangers of Grapefruit Juice

Grapefruit juice has long been known to alter the effects of certain medications, but not all doctors warn their patients about these potential dangers.*

Grapefruit juice contains compounds that inhibit an important enzyme called CYP3A4, which is found in the liver and intestines. CYP3A4 is one of several enzymes that help break down up to 70% of all medications.

Grapefruit juice that is made from concentrate usually contains the entire fruit, including the rind—the primary source of the compound that affects drug metabolism. Grapefruit juice that is not made from concentrate contains less of this compound. However, to be safe, it's best to avoid grapefruit juice (and grapefruit itself) altogether if you take certain medications.

Among the drugs that can interact with grapefruit juice…

•**Antiarrhythmic medications,** such as *amiodarone* (Cordarone), *quinidine* and *disopyramide* (Norpace), which are taken for abnormal heart rhythms.

Risks: Heart arrhythmias as well as thyroid, pulmonary or liver damage.

•**Blood pressure–lowering calcium channel blockers,** such as *felodipine, nifedipine* (Procardia) and *verapamil* (Calan).

Risks: A precipitous drop in blood pressure, as well as flushing, swelling of the extremities, headaches, irregular heartbeat and, in rare cases, heart attack.

•**Cholesterol-lowering drugs,** such as *atorvastatin* (Lipitor), *lovastatin* (Mevacor) and *simvastatin* (Zocor).

Risks: Headache, stomach upset, liver inflammation and muscle pain or weakness.

•**Sedatives** such as *diazepam* (Valium) and *triazolam* (Halcion).

Risks: Dizziness, confusion and drowsiness.

*As a general guideline, it is best not to drink any juice at the same time that you take medication. Instead, use water to swallow pills.

Dangers of Apple Juice and Orange Juice

Researchers found that apple, orange and grapefruit juice decrease the absorption of...

- Allergy medication *fexofenadine* (Allegra).
- Antibiotics, such as *ciprofloxacin* (Cipro) and *levofloxacin* (Levaquin).
- Antifungal drug *itraconazole* (Sporanox).
- Blood pressure–lowering beta-blockers, such as *atenolol* (Tenormin).
- Chemotherapy drug *etoposide* (Toposar).

If you are taking any of these drugs, it is probably safe to drink apple or orange juice (and eat whole fruits) at least two hours before or three hours after taking the medications. Check with your doctor first. Avoid grapefruit juice (and grapefruit itself) altogether.

Dangers of Coffee

Do not drink coffee at the same time that you take any medication. *Limit daily consumption of coffee to one to two cups if you take...*

- **Antacids.** Because coffee contains acid, it counteracts the effectiveness of OTC antacids such as calcium carbonate (TUMS) and Maalox.
- **Aspirin or other nonsteroidal anti-inflammatory (NSAID) medications,** such as *ibuprofen* (Advil) or *naproxen* (Aleve). Because coffee increases stomach acidity, combining it with these drugs may increase risk for gastro-intestinal side effects, including stomach irritation and bleeding.
- **Bronchodilator *theophylline*** (Elixophyllin), used to treat asthma or emphysema. Consuming coffee with the bronchodilator can slow the breakdown of the drug, leading to higher blood levels and an increased risk for nausea, vomiting, palpitations and seizures.
- **Monoamine oxidase inhibitor (MAOI) antidepressants,** such as *phenelzine* (Nardil) and *selegiline* (Eldepryl). The combination may increase anxiety.
- **Osteoporosis drug *alendronate*** (Fosamax). Studies show that coffee (and orange juice) can inhibit absorption of Fosamax by 60%.

Dangers of Cranberry Juice

In the United Kingdom, there have been at least eight recent reports of bleeding in patients (one of whom died) after they drank cranberry juice with the blood-thinning medication *warfarin* (Coumadin).

Health officials were unable to definitively link the bleeding to the combination of cranberry juice and warfarin, but it's probably safest to avoid cranberry juice altogether if you're taking this medication. If you take another drug with blood-thinning effects, such as aspirin, you can probably drink cranberry juice occasionally (no more than four ounces—at least two hours before or three hours after taking the medication). Consult your doctor.

Danger of Milk

The calcium in milk can interact with certain medications. *Drink milk at least two hours before or three hours after taking...*

•**Antacids,** such as calcium carbonate products (Rolaids) or sodium bicarbonate products (Alka-Seltzer and Brioschi). Drinking milk with these antacids can cause milk-alkali syndrome, a condition characterized by high blood calcium levels that can lead to kidney stones or even kidney failure.

•**Antibiotics,** such as tetracyclines and *ciprofloxacin* (Cipro). Calcium blocks absorption of these drugs, decreasing their effectiveness. Calcium-fortified juices are believed to have the same effect.

Better Drug Metabolism

Our bodies need nutrients to properly metabolize most medications. Chief among these nutrients is protein. Though we tend to eat less protein as we age—due to a variety of reasons, such as dental problems that make it harder to chew meat—we actually require more of this nutrient, since our bodies become less efficient at digesting and utilizing it.

Because the lining of the small and large intestines—where drugs are absorbed—regenerates every three to seven days, you need a continual supply of protein to maintain healthy levels of the enzymes that promote metabolism of medications.

To facilitate drug metabolism: Aim to eat about half a gram of protein daily for every pound of body weight.

Good sources: Fish, meats, eggs, peanut butter and soybeans.

B vitamins also play a key role in drug metabolism. Food sources rich in B vitamins include meats, fortified cereals, bananas and oatmeal.

Helpful: If you skip breakfast and aren't much of a meat eater, consider taking a multivitamin supplement containing the recommended daily intake of B vitamins.

CHAPTER 9

Healthful Eyes, Ears, Nose and Mouth

Save Your Sight

Jeffrey R. Anshel, OD, founder of the Ocular Nutrition Society. He is author of *What You Must Know About Food and Supplements for Optimal Vision Care: Ocular Nutrition Handbook.* EStreetEyes.com

Vision problems in the US have increased at alarming rates, including a 19% increase in cataracts and a 25% increase in macular degeneration since 2000.

Why the increase? Americans are living longer, and eyes with a lot of mileage are more likely to break down. But not getting the right nutrients plays a big role, too—and the right foods and supplements can make a big difference.

Of course, people with eye symptoms or a diagnosed eye disease should work closely with their doctors. I also recommend medical supervision for people who are taking multiple supplements.

But here are common eye problems and the foods and supplements that can fight them…

Dry Eyes

The eyes naturally get drier with age, but dry-eye syndrome—a chronic problem with the quantity and quality of tears—often is due to nutritional deficiencies. Poor nutrition can permit damaging free radicals to accumulate in the glands that produce tears.

What to do: Take one-half teaspoon of cod liver oil twice a week. It's an excellent source of DHA (docosahexaenoic acid, an omega-3 fatty acid) and vitamins A and D, nutrients that improve the quality of tears and help them lubricate more effectively.

Also helpful: BioTears, an oral supplement that includes curcumin and other eye-protecting ingredients. (I am on the scientific advisory board of BioSyntrx, which makes BioTears and Eye & Body Complete, see next page, but I have no financial interest in the company.) I have found improvement in about 80% of patients who take BioTears. Follow the directions on the label.

Cataracts

Cataracts typically are caused by the age-related clumping of proteins in the crystalline lens of the eyes. More than half of Americans will have cataracts by the time they're 80.

What to do: Eat spinach, kale and other dark leafy greens every day. They contain lutein, an antioxidant that reduces the free-radical damage that increases cataract risk. (Lutein and zeaxanthin, another antioxidant, are the only carotenoids that concentrate in the lenses of the eyes.)

Important: Cook kale or other leafy greens with a little bit of oil…or eat them with a meal that contains olive oil or other fats. The carotenoids are fat-soluble, so they require a little fat for maximal absorption.

I also advise patients to take 500 milligrams (mg) of vitamin C three or four times a day (cut back if you get diarrhea). One study found that those who took vitamin C supplements for 10 years were 64% less likely to have cataracts.

The supplement Eye & Body Complete contains a mix of eye-protecting compounds, including bioflavonoids, bilberry and vitamins A and D. Follow instructions on the label.

Computer Vision Syndrome

The National Institute of Occupational Safety and Health reports that 88% of people who work at a computer for more than three hours a day complain of computer-related problems, including blurred vision, headaches, neck pain and eye dryness.

What to do: Take a supplement that contains about 6 mg of astaxanthin, a carotenoid. It reduces eyestrain by improving the stamina of eye muscles.

Also helpful: The 20/20/20 rule. After every 20 minutes on a computer, take 20 seconds and look 20 feet away.

Reduced Night Vision

True night blindness (nyctalopia) is rare in the US, but many older adults find that they struggle to see at night, which can make night driving difficult.

What to do: Take a daily supplement that includes one-half mg of copper and 25 mg of zinc. Zinc deficiencies have been associated with poor night vision—and you'll need the extra copper to "balance" the zinc. Zinc helps the body produce vitamin A, which is required by the retina to detect light.

Also helpful: The foods for AMD (below).

Age-Related Macular Degeneration (AMD)

This serious disease is the leading cause of blindness in older adults. Most people with AMD first will notice that their vision has become slightly hazy. As the disease progresses, it can cause a large blurred area in the center of the field of vision.

What to do: Eat several weekly servings of spinach or other brightly colored vegetables, such as kale and yellow peppers, or egg yolks. The nutrients and antioxidants in these foods can help slow the progression of AMD. The National Eye Institute's Age-Related Eye Disease Study (AREDS) reported that patients who already had macular degeneration and had adequate intakes of beta-carotene, zinc, copper and vitamins C and E were 25% less likely to develop an advanced form of the disease.

Also helpful: The Eye & Body Complete supplement, mentioned earlier. It contains all of the ingredients used in the original AREDS study—plus many others, including generous amounts of lutein and zeaxanthin that were included in a follow-up study, known as AREDS2—and was found to have positive effects.

Exercises to Improve Eye Strength

Marc Grossman, OD, LAc, holistic developmental/behavioral optometrist, licensed acupuncturist and medical director, Natural Eye Care, New Paltz, New York. He is coauthor of *Greater Vision and Natural Eye Care.* NaturalEyeCare.com

When it comes to signs of aging, different people have different pet peeves. Some of us really don't like those gray hairs…others sigh over a lost silhouette…still others hate needing reading glasses to see what's on the menu.

Since exercise improves the strength, flexibility and function of our bodies, it makes sense that eye exercises could improve our ability to see close up. Yet this is a controversial topic. Though various studies have found no clear benefit from eye exercises, many holistic practitioners and their patients say that vision can indeed be improved.

The challenge with aging eyes: Many people first become farsighted—meaning that nearby objects look blurry even though more distant objects are clear—starting in their 40s. This is due to presbyopia, a condition in which the aging lens of the eye becomes too stiff to focus clearly up close.

Detractors of eye exercise say that it won't restore lens elasticity. But that's not the point. Eye exercises can improve the strength, flexibility and adaptability of muscles that control eye movement and encourage a mental focus that helps the brain and eyes work better together. This can slow the progression of farsightedness and possibly improve vision.

So can eye exercises help us say good riddance to reading glasses? The answer is yes for some people—and it certainly can't hurt to try.

The four exercises below will help you improve close-up vision. While you do the exercises, remember to keep breathing and keep blinking. And smile! Smiling reduces tension, which helps your muscles work optimally and your brain focus on what's around you.

Try to do the exercises while not wearing any reading glasses—or if your close-up vision is not good enough for that, wear weaker reading glasses than you normally do. If you usually wear glasses or contacts for distance vision, it is OK to wear those while doing the exercises.

How long to practice: Do each exercise for three to four minutes, for a total practice time of about 15 minutes per session, at least three times weekly. If you get headaches while exercising your eyes, reduce the time spent on each exercise—and see your eye doctor if the problem persists.

•**Letter reading**—for better scanning accuracy and conscious eye control when reading or using a computer.

Preparation: Type up a chart with four rows of random letters, just large enough that you can read them while holding the page at a typical reading distance (type size will vary depending on an individual's vision). Leave space between each row. In row one, type all capitals, one space in between each letter...row two, all lowercase, one space in between each letter...row three, all lowercase, no spaces...row four, wordlike groups of random letters arranged as if in a sentence.

Exercise: Hold the chart with both hands. Looking at row one, read each letter aloud left to right, then right to left. Then read every second letter... then every third letter. If your mind wanders, start over.

Over time: When you master row one, try the same techniques with row two...then row three...then row four. If you find that you have memorized parts of the chart, make a new one using different letters.

•**Near and far**—for improved focus and focusing speed when switching your gaze from close objects to distant objects (such as when checking gauges on a car as you drive).

Preparation: Type a chart with six to eight rows of random capital letters, each letter about one-half inch tall (or as tall as necessary for you to read them from 10 feet away). Tack the chart to a wall and stand back 10 feet.

Exercise: Hold a pencil horizontally, with its embossed letters facing you, about six inches from your nose (or as close as possible without it looking blurry). Read any letter on the pencil, then read any letter on the chart. Keep doing this, switching back and forth as fast as you can without letting the letters blur.

Over time: Do this with one eye covered, then the other.

•**Pencil pushups**—to promote eye teamwork. All you need is a pencil.

Exercise: Hold a pencil horizontally at eye level 12 inches from your face (or as far as necessary to see the pencil clearly). With both eyes, look at one particular letter on the pencil...keep looking while bringing the pencil closer to your face. If the letter blurs or doubles, it means that one eye is no longer accurately on target—so move the pencil back until the letter is clear once more...then try again to slowly bring the pencil closer while keeping the letter in focus.

•**The "hot dog"**—for improved flexibility of the muscles within the eye that allow the lens to change shape. No props are needed.

Exercise: With your hands at chest height about eight inches in front of you, point your index fingers and touch the tips together, so that your index fingers are horizontal. Gaze at any target in the distance and, without changing your focus, raise your fingers into your line of sight. Notice that a "mini hot dog" has appeared between the tips of your fingers. Still gazing at the distant object, pull your fingertips apart slightly—and observe that the hot dog is now floating in the air. Keep the hot dog there for two breaths... then look directly at your fingers for two breaths, noticing that the hot dog disappears. Look again at the distant object and find the hot dog once again. Continue switching your gaze back and forth every two breaths.

As your close-up vision improves, you may find that you need less-powerful reading glasses—or none at all—for your day-to-day activities.

Nutrients That Reverse Cataracts

Marc Grossman, OD, LAc, holistic developmental/behavioral optometrist, licensed acupuncturist and medical director, Natural Eye Care, New Paltz, New York. He is coauthor of *Greater Vision and Natural Eye Care*. NaturalEyeCare.com

Are cataracts no big deal? Cataract surgery has become so quick and effective that many people now ignore opportunities to protect themselves from getting cataracts in the first place. They assume that their eyes can be made good as new one day with some simple surgery—so why worry about it now?

Please don't think that way. While cataract surgery has been well perfected, there is always potential for problems—including retinal detachment. The good news is that there are very simple ways to ward off the cloudiness of cataracts.

Cataracts begin forming in the eyes shortly after you pass the age of 50 and currently affect some 22.3 million Americans. One of the keys to cataract prevention is a combination of diet and supplements that boost the body's level of glutathione, a powerful antioxidant that is distinguished by its ability to interfere with the development of cataracts.

Several studies show that glutathione can prevent the further formation of cataracts and in my own experience, I've seen glutathione reverse the development of cataracts that have already formed. That's pretty extraordinary.

A Closer Look

To appreciate how glutathione works, it's important to understand how cataracts develop. The lenses in your eyes are made up of proteins arranged in a very orderly way so that light passes easily through them. But as we age—especially if we lapse into poor diets, smoking or too much alcohol or develop diabetes or other chronic diseases—oxygen interacts with these proteins, creating highly reactive free radicals that cause the proteins to clump together. As they do, it becomes more difficult for light to pass through the lenses, and the result is cataracts and vision that's increasingly blurry.

Here's where antioxidants come into play. These substances can protect cells against the effects of free radicals. Vitamins A, C and E are antioxidants that we all know about. Those that are somewhat less well known include beta-carotene, lutein, lycopene and selenium. All of these help to slow the development of cataracts, but when it comes to the eye lens, the most powerful antioxidant is glutathione.

If glutathione—which is made up of three amino acids (cysteine, glycine, glutamic acid)—were easy for the body to absorb, preventing cataracts would be a simple matter of taking regular supplements. Unfortunately, we have the opposite scenario—glutathione is far more difficult to absorb than the more familiar antioxidants.

The solution is twofold. First, eat foods that boost your body's ability to create glutathione, primarily in your liver. The list includes asparagus, eggs, broccoli, avocados, garlic, onions, cantaloupe, watermelon, spinach and strawberries. However, it's doubtful that diet alone can raise glutathione to sufficient levels for preventing the formation of cataracts. I also suggest that you eliminate, or at least reduce, the amount of refined sugar in your diet (including milk sugar, which is found in dairy products) and take supplements, not of glutathione itself but of substances known to encourage production of the body's level of glutathione—N-acetyl cysteine (NAC), alpha lipoic acid and vitamin C. Alpha lipoic acid is particularly effective. You can buy it and NAC at some drugstores, many health-food outlets and online. One brand is DeTox Formula made by Vital Nutrients (800-383-6008, PureFormulas.com).

NAC and alpha lipoic acid are generally OK for everyone as long as the safe dosage is not exceeded—up to 300 mg for alpha lipoic acid and up to 600 mg for NAC. However, it's best to talk to your doctor before taking either supplement, because they may lower thyroid hormone levels, adversely affect people with certain kidney conditions as well as strengthen the effects of certain medications—including ACE inhibitors for high blood pressure and immunosuppressive drugs.

Ultraviolet light encourages the proteins in the lens to clump together. So in addition to increasing levels of glutathione by eating the foods above and taking supplements, be sure to wear quality sunglasses that block UV light and a wide-brimmed hat whenever you're out on a sunny day.

Prevent Glaucoma with a Folate Supplement

Study titled "A Prospective Study of Folate, Vitamin B-6, and Vitamin B-12 Intake in Relation to Exfoliation Glaucoma or Suspected Exfoliation Glaucoma," published in *JAMA Ophthalmology*.

Glaucoma is an insidious disease—literally happening before your very eyes undetected, having virtually no symptoms until, in a blink, you've got eye surgery on your plate and you may even be going blind. You may think that, nowadays, glaucoma is easily treatable, but one form of glaucoma, pseudoexfoliation glaucoma (called "PEX" or sometimes just exfoliation glaucoma) is much harder to fix than others. Research from Harvard Medical School, though, is showing that the more folate you get each day, the less likely PEX will develop.

Are You at Risk?

PEX is caused by pressurized buildup of debris that clogs the eye's ability to drain, and it can lead to cataract formation, destruction of the optic nerve and blindness. PEX can happen because it's in your genes or because your eyes have been exposed to too much of the sun's ultraviolet (UV) light. People who live in some northern parts of the world, such as Scandinavia (possibly because of genes) and higher altitudes (where the thin air encourages more UV-radiation exposure) are also more at risk for this eye disease. People with PEX also have high levels of an amino acid called homocysteine in their blood, tears and eye fluid. Because B vitamins can help keep homocysteine levels in check, some researchers thought that getting enough B vitamins was the key, but the team from Harvard Medical School discovered that it's not quite that simple— it appears that you must get a certain B vitamin in a certain specific way.

Uncovering the Precise Nutritional Link

To get a clearer picture, the Harvard researchers analyzed information from about 120,000 people from two very large, long-term health study databases, the Nurses' Health Study and the Health Professionals Follow-up Study, with a specific focus on people who were 40 years old or older, were free of glaucoma at the start of the study, had had eye exams within a certain two-year period and had provided information about their dietary habits. They discovered that people who ultimately got PEX were deficient in one particular B vitamin, folate. They also found that, although the amount of folate gotten only from food had little impact on prevention of PEX, getting enough from a supplement made a big difference.

Folate Is an Eye-Saver

People with the highest intake of folate—at least 335 micrograms (mcg) per day for women and 434 mcg for men—from vitamin supplements had an 83% reduced risk of PEX compared with people who did not take such supplements. The good news is that any high-quality B complex vitamin supplement, which will generally contain 400 mcg of folate, together with a diet rich in green leafy vegetables, fortified whole grains, beans and peas and especially beef liver (if you have a taste for it) will supply you with enough folate to protect you from PEX. You can even find folate supplements that contain 800 mcg or more, but be aware that the daily tolerable upper limit of supplemental folate for adults, according to the Institute of Medicine, is 1,000 mcg. Also, be aware that folate supplements can interfere with the anticancer effectiveness of the drug *methotrexate*. Speak with your doctor if you take that drug. Folate supplements also aren't well absorbed in people taking antiepileptic drugs or *sulfasalazine* (Azulfidine, used to treat ulcerative colitis), so guidance about folate supplement dosage, in these instances, also should be discussed with a doctor.

We're increasingly being told by medical experts to ditch vitamin supplements and get our nutrients from whole foods. Although I think this is generally sound advice over pill-popping, even if those pills are vitamins, I also think it's important to pay heed to studies like this one that show that a supplement is exactly what's needed to stave off a serious condition. And sight-robbing glaucoma is serious enough in anyone's book!

How to Slow, Stop and Perhaps Even Reverse Vision-Robbing Macular Degeneration

Stephen Rose, PhD, chief research officer of the Foundation Fighting Blindness. Dr. Rose is the former director of the Division of Clinical Recombinant DNA Research at the Office of Biotechnology Activities of the National Institutes of Health. Blindness.org

Age-related macular degeneration (AMD), the most common cause of vision loss in people over age 55, has always been considered a difficult—if not impossible—condition to treat.

Now: There is more reason than ever before to be hopeful that this dreaded eye disease, which affects about 10 million Americans, can be slowed, stopped or even reversed.

Exciting new scientific findings...

Breakthroughs for Dry AMD

Dry AMD, which affects about 90% of people with AMD, occurs when the light-sensitive cells in the macula slowly break down, gradually blurring central vision—which is necessary for reading and driving.

There is no treatment for dry AMD, though many drugs are in clinical trials. In the meantime, we now have evidence that certain nutrients can help control the disease, and exciting advances are taking place in stem cell therapy.

•**Nutrients that can help.** The Age-Related Eye Disease Study (AREDS), landmark research conducted by the National Eye Institute, found that a supplement containing high levels of antioxidants and zinc reduced the risk for advanced dry and wet AMD (the latest stages of AMD) in people with vision loss in one or both eyes.

The daily regimen: 500 mg of vitamin C...400 international units (IU) of vitamin E...15 mg of beta-carotene...80 mg of zinc...and 2 mg of copper. People with all stages of AMD were studied. With early-stage AMD, there may be no symptoms or vision loss. The condition is detected when an eye-care professional can see drusen (yellow deposits under the retina) during a dilated eye exam.

Scientists also are studying other nutrients for dry AMD, and there have been several positive reports. *For example...*

•**Zeaxanthin and lutein.** When 60 people with mild-to-moderate dry AMD took 8 mg a day of zeaxanthin for one year, they reported a marked improvement in vision (more "visual acuity" and a "sharpening of detailed high-contrast discrimination") along with visual restoration of some blind spots, researchers reported in the journal *Optometry.* A group receiving 9 mg of lutein daily along with zeaxanthin also had improvements in vision.

Many supplements that contain all of the nutrients mentioned earlier are available over-the-counter (OTC). But these should not be taken without a diagnosis of large drusen and monitoring by a doctor—some of these nutrients could be harmful for certain individuals, such as current and former smokers.

•**Stem cell therapy.** Perhaps one of the most remarkable findings ever reported in the literature of AMD treatment occurred earlier this year when new retinal cells grown from stem cells were used to restore some of the eyesight of a 78-year-old woman who was nearly blind due to a very advanced form of dry AMD.

The breakthrough therapy involved the use of human embryonic stem cells, which are capable of producing any of the more than 200 types of specialized cells in the body. New retinal cells grown from stem cells were injected into the patient's retina. Four months later, the patient had not lost any additional vision and, in fact, her vision seemed to improve slightly.

For more information: Go to ClinicalTrials.gov and search "advanced dry age-related macular degeneration and stem cells."

Breakthroughs for Wet AMD

Wet AMD, which affects about 10% of people with AMD, is more severe than the early and intermediate stages of the dry form. It occurs when abnormal blood vessels behind the retina start to grow. This causes blood and fluid to leak from the vessels, and the macula to swell. Because the condition progresses quickly, it requires prompt treatment for the best chance of saving your vision. You are at an increased risk for wet AMD if you have dry AMD in one or both eyes...or you have wet AMD in one eye (the other eye is at risk).

The two standard treatments for wet AMD are the injection of a medication directly into the eye to block the growth of the abnormal blood vessels...and photodynamic therapy, in which a drug that's injected into the arm flows to the abnormal blood vessels in the eye and is activated there by a laser beam that destroys the vessels.

What's new...

•**More affordable drug choice.** The drugs *ranibizumab* (Lucentis) and *bevacizumab* (Avastin), which are injected into the eye, halt or reverse vision loss. However, these drugs have a huge price disparity. Lucentis, which is FDA-approved as a treatment for wet AMD, costs $2,000 per injection, while Avastin, a cancer drug that is used "off-label" to treat AMD, costs $50.

New finding: In a two-year study, both drugs worked equally well, with two-thirds of patients having "driving vision" (20/40 or better).

Another option: Aflibercept (Eylea), also injected into the eye, was approved by the FDA for wet AMD in November 2011. Research shows that every-other-month injections of Eylea (about $1,800 per injection) can be as effective as monthly injections of Lucentis.

Bottom line: You now have three safe and effective AMD treatment options to discuss with your doctor.

•**At-home monitoring.** Monthly monitoring by an ophthalmologist or optometrist for the subtle visual changes that herald wet AMD (or indicate a diagnosed case is worsening) is impractical for many.

New: An at-home system, the ForeseeHome AMD Monitoring Program, was recently approved by the FDA. You look into this lightweight and portable monitor for a few minutes daily. If results indicate a problem, you and your doctor are alerted to schedule an eye appointment.

What Is Macular Degeneration?

Age-related macular degeneration (AMD) causes progressive damage to the macula, the part of the eye that allows us to see objects clearly. With "dry" AMD, there is a thinning of the macula, which gradually blurs central vision but generally does not cause a total loss of sight. With "wet" AMD, a more severe form of the disease, abnormal blood vessels grow beneath the macula, leaking fluid and blood. Wet AMD often progresses rapidly, leading to significant vision loss or even blindness.

Surprising Ways to Improve Your Hearing

Michael Seidman, MD, director of the Otolaryngology Research Laboratory and the Division of Otologic/Neurotologic Surgery at the Henry Ford Health System in Detroit. Dr. Seidman is coauthor, with Marie Moneysmith, of *Save Your Hearing Now.*

Aside from protecting your ears from blasting stereos and jackhammers, there's not much you can do to control what happens to your hearing, right? Wrong!

It's true that genetic and environmental factors (such as loud noises) are usually what cause hearing loss. But most people have far more ability to prevent hearing loss—or even improve their hearing—than they realize.

Here's why: Most problems with hearing begin when the hair cells located in the cochlea, or inner ear, don't work well or stop functioning and die. Improving blood supply to the inner ear and tamping down inflammation within the body are among the strategies that may help keep your hearing sharp.

At first glance, you wouldn't think that the steps below would have anything to do with your hearing. But they have a lot to do with it.

Here's my advice for improving your hearing or keeping it intact…

Check Your Meds

If you're having trouble hearing, see an otolaryngologist (ear, nose and throat specialist) or audiologist for an evaluation—and ask your doctor about the medications you take. *Among the many medications that are "ototoxic"—that is, they can lead to hearing loss…*

•**Antidepressants** such as *fluoxetine* (Prozac) and *amitriptyline.*

•**Antibiotics,** such as *erythromycin, gentamicin* and *tetracycline.*

•**Nonsteroidal anti-inflammatory drugs (NSAIDs),** such as aspirin and *ibuprofen* (Motrin).

If medication is causing your hearing loss, stopping the drug or switching to a new one, under your doctor's supervision, may improve your hearing.

For a list of drugs that can cause hearing loss: Go to the hearing loss resource website, NVRC.org (click on Hearing Loss, then Ototoxic Drugs for a downloadable PDF).

Get the Right Nutrients

Certain nutrients are known to promote blood flow and help fight inflammation throughout the body—including in the ears.

To ensure that you have adequate levels of such nutrients, consider taking targeted supplements to protect your hearing. Among those that are beneficial are alpha lipoic acid, acetyl-L-carnitine, L-glutathione and CoQ10. Taking these supplements may help slow hearing loss and protect against damage from loud noises.

What to do: To determine which supplements (including doses) are best for you, consult an integrative physician. To find one near you, contact the Academy of Integrative Health and Medicine at AIHM.org.

Look at Your Lifestyle

Other ways to increase your odds of keeping your hearing sharp as long as possible…

•**Chill out.** If you're late for a meeting and stuck in traffic, your stress levels will probably climb. But what's that got to do with your hearing? Quite a lot, actually.

Common Vitamin Protects Against Hearing Loss

In an 18-year study of 51,529 men, those age 60 and older with the highest intake of the B vitamin folate (folic acid) had a 21% lower risk for hearing loss than men of the same age who consumed the least folate.

To protect your hearing: Eat folate-rich foods, such as spinach, chickpeas, sunflower seeds and fortified cereals, daily.

Caution: Consuming more than 800 mcg of folate daily has been linked to higher risk for colon cancer. Researchers do not know why folate appears to protect hearing nor whether the nutrient would help prevent hearing loss in women.

Josef Shargorodsky, MD, otolaryngologist, Massachusetts Eye and Ear Infirmary, Boston.

Research has now shown that brain chemicals called dynorphins respond to stress by triggering inflammation in the brain—and in the inner ear. Inflammation not only exacerbates hearing loss but also hearing-related problems such as tinnitus.

What to do: Setting aside time each day for anything that alleviates tension—be it daily meditation, yoga or listening to restful music—may reduce your stress levels…and improve your hearing or help prevent hearing loss.

Surprising new research: Chewing gum may curb hearing loss in some cases—perhaps by distracting the brain from stress that may be interfering with the brain's processing of sound.

•**Keep off the pounds.** Evidence is continuing to mount that the more a person is overweight, the greater his/her risk for hearing loss. What's the link? Factors closely related to obesity, such as high blood pressure, are believed to restrict blood flow to the inner ear.

What to do: Both men and women should aim for a body mass index (BMI) of 18.5 to 24.9.

•**Get enough exercise.** In recent research, women who walked at least two hours a week had a 15% lower risk for hearing loss, compared with those who walked less than one hour a week. The hearing protection conferred by exercise is also believed to apply to men.

What to do: To protect your hearing—and perhaps even improve it—spend at least two hours a week doing exercise, such as brisk walking.

•**Avoid cigarette smoke.** Smoking is bad for the lungs, the heart and many other parts of the body. But the ears? Absolutely! In a study of adults ages 48 to 92, smokers were more likely than nonsmokers to have hearing impairment. And though it's not well known, even nonsmokers who live with smokers (this includes cigar and pipe smokers, too) are more likely to have hearing loss, suggesting that secondhand smoke can cause damage that impairs hearing.

What to do: Kick the tobacco habit—and encourage family members to do the same.

Getting Enough Zs

Sleep apnea, a disorder marked by chronic breathing pauses during sleep, has been recently linked to a 90% increased risk for low-frequency hearing loss (difficulty hearing conversation on the phone is a hallmark) and a 31% increased risk for high-frequency hearing loss (this often makes it hard to understand higher-pitched sounds, such as a woman's voice).

The results are preliminary, but some researchers believe that sleep apnea may trigger hearing loss due to poor blood flow to the cochlea, or inner ear.

What to do: If you snore (a common symptom of sleep apnea), see a doctor to determine whether you have sleep apnea and ask whether you should also have your hearing tested. If you have sleep apnea, it's possible that treating it will improve your hearing.

Don't Feel Ready for a Hearing Aid?

Barbara E. Weinstein, PhD, a professor of audiology and head of the Audiology Program at The City University of New York Graduate Center, where she specializes in hearing loss in older adults, hearing screening, disability assessment and evidence-based practice. She is the author of the textbook *Geriatric Audiology.*

If you are reluctant (or can't afford) to use a hearing aid, there are dozens of personal sound amplification products (PSAPs), over-the-counter devices that can help you hear a little better but don't cost as much as hearing aids, which run up to $3,000 each.

Not Quite a Hearing Aid

Hearing aids are recommended for those who have been diagnosed with hearing loss by an audiologist. PSAPs, which come in many shapes and sizes, often resembling a Bluetooth headset, are meant to amplify sounds in situations where hearing is difficult, such as large gatherings or noisy restaurants.

In reality, it's not an either-or choice. Only 20% to 25% of people who could benefit from a hearing aid actually use one. PSAPs, with their lower price and availability on the Internet and in pharmacies can serve as "training wheels" for people who want to hear better but hesitate to shell out big bucks for a hearing aid.

Important: The hearing aids sold by audiologists are approved by the FDA as medical devices and must meet certain standards related, for example, to frequency ranges and distortion. PSAPs, on the other hand, are classified as electronic products. They aren't subject to FDA review, so you can't assume that they'll work for you. However, some PSAPs already rival the quality of "official" hearing aids and will keep getting better as technology improves.

Know What You Need

Before you look into PSAPs, get tested by an audiologist. About 14% of adults in their 50s, one-quarter in their 60s and more than one-third of those age 65 and older have some degree of age-related hearing loss. But do not assume that your hearing is normal—or that hearing loss is inevitable.

You may think that your hearing is becoming impaired because of your age when, in fact, it may be due to a medical issue, such as infection, abnormal bone growth, an inner-ear tumor or even earwax—all of which can be treated and sometimes reversed.

If your hearing loss is not related to a medical issue, a PSAP may be appropriate in the following situations...

•**You have trouble hearing the TV.** It is a common complaint but fairly easy to overcome. Inexpensive earbuds or a headset that merely amplifies the sound may be all that you need. Some products are wireless or have long cords that plug directly into the TV.

•**You have trouble hearing in quiet environments.** Speech can sound muffled or be entirely unintelligible if you have age-related hearing loss. Even if you can easily hear background sounds (such as music), you might struggle with the high-frequency sounds that are characteristic of speech.

If you plan to use a PSAP mainly at home or in other quiet settings (such as a museum or a hushed restaurant), look for a device that amplifies high frequencies more than low ones. You'll hear voices more clearly without being overwhelmed by the volume of sounds.

Warning: Some inexpensive products boost both high and low frequencies indiscriminately—avoid them. Your best choice will be a product that allows you to make adjustments and fine-tune it in different settings.

•**You have trouble hearing in noisy environments.** Even mild hearing loss can make it hard to hear voices over the din of clattering plates, a chattering crowd and background music. A simple amplifier won't work because it will make all of the sounds louder.

Better: A device that amplifies the sounds you want to hear while filtering out the rest. Look for a PSAP that has a directional microphone that will pick up speech while muting noise…noise cancellation to filter out low-frequency background sounds…volume control…and multiple channels that are suitable for different sound environments.

•**You're on the fence.** It's common for people to put off getting a hearing aid because of embarrassment or cost. (Hearing aids aren't covered by Medicare or most insurance plans.) You might be telling yourself, "Maybe I'll get one when I'm a lot older."

Important: Don't wait too long. The parts of the brain associated with hearing become less active when they aren't used. You need to hear sounds to keep this brain circuitry working and actively processing speech.

You might want to use a PSAP while you're making up your mind about hearing aids. Even if you get a PSAP that just boosts volume, it will keep the brain signals firing. In my opinion, it's reasonable to use one of these devices for a few months or even a few years. You can always buy a hearing aid later.

Hearing Aid Bargains

Jim Miller, an advocate for older Americans, writes "Savvy Senior," a weekly information column syndicated in more than 400 newspapers nationwide. Based in Norman, Oklahoma, he also offers a free senior e-news service at SavvySenior.org.

Hearing aids have become very expensive. But you can reduce or even eliminate the cost…

•**Hearing aid bargains.** Most Costco stores sell top brands of hearing aids for 30% to 50% less than other warehouse chains, hearing aid dealers and audiologist offices. They offer high-quality devices under the brands Kirkland Signature (the Costco house brand), Rexton, ReSound, Bernafon and Phonak at prices ranging from $500 to $1,800 per ear. This includes an in-store hearing test, fitting by a specialist and follow-up care.

Also, websites including EmbraceHearing.com and Audicus.com sell high-quality hearing aids directly from the manufacturer for as little as $400 or $500. But you will need to get a hearing evaluation from a local audiologist first, which can cost between $50 and $250.

•**Check your insurance.** Most private health insurers don't cover hearing aids, but a few do. UnitedHealthcare, for example, offers custom-programmed hearing aids through hiHealthInnovations (hiHealthInnovations.com) for

Fish Reduces Risk for Age-Related Hearing Loss

People over age 50 who eat at least two five-ounce servings of fish per week have a 42% lower risk of developing hearing loss, compared with people who eat less than one serving of fish per week.

Possible reason: Omega-3s may help preserve circulation in the inner ear. Fish that are high in omega-3 fatty acids, such as salmon, sardines and mackerel, provide the greatest benefit.

Paul Mitchell, MD, professor, department of ophthalmology, University of Sydney, Australia, and coauthor of a study of 2,956 people, published in *American Journal of Clinical Nutrition.*

$599 to $899 each to people enrolled in its employer-sponsored individual or vision plans.

Some other insurers contribute a specified amount toward hearing aids, typically $500 or $1,000, or give a discount if you purchase hearing aids from a contracted provider.

Three states—Arkansas, New Hampshire and Rhode Island—require insurers to cover hearing aid costs for adults, and 20 states require it for children. Eligibility and amounts vary by state, and certain insurance plans are exempt.

Original Medicare (Parts A and B) and Medigap supplemental policies do not cover hearing aids, but some Medicare Advantage (Part C) plans, which are obtained through private insurers, include hearing aids. To find a plan that covers hearing aids, call 800-633-4227 or go to Medicare.gov/find-a-plan.

If you are a current or retired federal employee or if a member of your family is enrolled in the Federal Employees Health Benefits Program, some insurers provide coverage, including a Blue Cross and Blue Shield plan that covers up to $2,500 every three years.

Medicaid programs in most states cover hearing aids. Contact your state's Medicaid program or visit Medicaid.gov.

•**Benefits for veterans.** The Department of Veterans Affairs provides hearing aids and replacement batteries free of charge to veterans if their hearing loss is connected to military service or linked to a medical condition treated at a VA hospital. Veterans also can get free hearing aids through the VA if hearing loss is severe enough to interfere with activities of daily life. Call 877-222-8387 or visit VA.gov.

Assistance programs: If your income is low, there are various programs that provide financial assistance for hearing aids. Check by calling your state vocational rehabilitation department (see Parac.org/svrp.html for contact information). Also contact Sertoma (Sertoma.org), a civic service organization that provides a list of state and national hearing aid assistance programs. Or call the National Institute on Deafness and Other Communication Disorders at 800-241-1044, and ask for a list of financial resources for hearing aids.

How Good Is Your Sense of Smell?

Jayant Pinto, MD, associate professor of otolaryngology–head and neck surgery in the department of surgery at The University of Chicago Medicine, where he specializes in sinus and nasal diseases and olfactory dysfunction.

Alan Hirsch, MD, founder and neurological director of the Smell & Taste Treatment and Research Foundation in Chicago. He is a neurologist and psychiatrist, and author of *Life's a Smelling Success.* SmellAndTaste.org

Can you smell the rose that's under your nose? What about the odor of burning toast? Or the foul smell of spoiled food?

Just as it's common to have fading vision or diminished hearing as you age, many people lose at least some of their ability to smell. In fact, about 25% of adults over the age of 53 have a reduced sense of smell, and the percentage rises to more than 60% in those age 80 and older.

An Early Alert

You're probably well aware that a decreased sense of smell can affect appetite. People who can't smell and/or taste their food tend to eat less and may suffer from weight loss or nutritional deficiencies. *But you might not know that a diminished sense of smell could also be an early indicator of a serious health problem…*

Surprising finding: In a recent study, people ranging from ages 57 to 85 who lost their ability to smell were more than three times more likely to die within five years than those with a normal sense of smell—the risk of dying was even higher than for individuals diagnosed with lung disease, heart failure or cancer.

This study didn't uncover the exact link between smelling loss and earlier-than-expected deaths. But the risk for neurodegenerative diseases could be a factor. It's also possible that *cellular senescence*, the age-related reduction in cell regeneration, affects the olfactory bulb or other parts of the olfactory system before it becomes apparent in other parts of the body.

Test Yourself

Even if you think your sense of smell is fine, some basic testing might show otherwise. In the study mentioned earlier, some individuals who thought they had a good sense of smell actually didn't, while some people who thought they had a problem with their sense of smell actually did well on the smell tests.

How to test yourself…

•**The alcohol test.** Hold an alcohol-swab packet near your belly button and open it up. If your sense of smell is perfect, you will detect the odor. If you can't smell it, raise it higher until you can. Some people won't detect the odor until it's just a few inches from the nose—or not even then. You can do the same test with anything that's strongly scented. The closer the item needs to be for you to smell it, the worse your sense of smell is.

•**Compare yourself to others.** Suspect that you have a problem if you're the only one in the family who doesn't notice the wonderful smell of brownies in the oven. Or if you say "Huh?" when your spouse mentions that the fireplace is smoking or that there's a nasty smell in the refrigerator.

If you think you have a diminished sense of smell: Get evaluated by an otolaryngologist or a neurologist. He/she can determine if your impairment is due to aging or a more serious problem that may have a better outcome if it is detected early.

What You Can Do

So far, a reduced sense of smell can't be restored.* *What can help...*

•**Practice smelling.** German scientists report that it may be possible to improve your sense of smell by smelling more. Spend a few minutes every day sniffing a variety of scents—spices, perfumes, aromatic foods, etc. This approach hasn't been proven, but it could be helpful for some people.

•**Eat a well-balanced diet and take a multivitamin,** which will provide the necessary micronutrients that help slow aging of the olfactory system and promote regeneration.

If you have appetite loss due to a reduced sense of smell...

•**Kick up the seasoning.** Food will not be very appealing if you can't smell or taste it. To make your dishes as flavorful and aromatic as possible, use plenty of strong spices, such as pepper, garlic, cilantro, ginger, etc., in your cooking.

•**Focus on preparation and presentation.**

Chefs have a saying: "The eyes eat first." Use brightly colored fruits and vegetables and other colorful ingredients, and add garnishes to your plate. Also, vary the textures of the foods you eat.

*Exception: If your loss of smell is due to nasal inflammation—from allergies, chronic sinusitis, etc.—intranasal steroid sprays and antihistamines may restore it.

Often, when the underlying problem is corrected, the sense of smell returns. People who quit smoking usually regain all or most of their sense of smell, but this can take years. *Also…*

•**The nutrients thiamine (100 milligrams daily) and phosphatidylcholine (9 grams daily) can elevate levels of neurotransmitters that improve the sense of smell.** In one study, about 40% of patients improved significantly after taking phosphatidylcholine for three months. The success rate with thiamine is somewhat lower.

•**Sniff therapy.** People who expose themselves to the same scent 20 to 50 times a day for several weeks will have an increase in scent receptors and will sometimes regain their ability to smell that particular scent.

Supplements That Help Prevent Gum Disease

Mark A. Breiner, DDS, an authority on holistic dentistry with a practice in Fairfield, Connecticut. Dr. Breiner is the author of *Whole-Body Dentistry: A Complete Guide to Understanding the Impact of Dentistry on Total Health.* WholeBodyDentistry.com

I f you're over age 65, the odds of getting gum disease jump to 64%. Even people who brush and floss and avoid sugar can fall victim because some risk factors (such as aging and having certain genes) are unavoidable. And as you know, oral health is connected with overall health—gum disease raises your risk for systemic health issues, such as stroke, diabetes and cancer. *Here are natural strategies you need to know…*

Keep Your Gums in the Pink

Here are natural ways to prevent and/or treat gum disease.

1. **Rinse with an herbal mouthwash.** Herbs such as echinacea, eucalyptus, lavender and thyme are good at killing harmful bacteria, so they help prevent gum disease and help heal gum tissue if gum disease has already developed. So look for a mouthwash that lists at least one of those herbs on the label (ideally all of them). While you're checking the ingredient list, make sure that the mouthwash is alcohol-free, because some studies have found an association between alcohol-based mouthwash and oral cancer. For example, you could try a brand called PerioWash (available online and in most drugstores) after

brushing and flossing each morning and night—it contains all four herbs mentioned above and no alcohol.

2. Take certain supplements.

•**Vitamin C.** Whether you have gum disease or not, ask your doctor about taking 500 milligrams (mg) daily of vitamin C because the nutrient builds collagen, a connective protein that is the foundation of gum tissue.

•**Coenzyme Q10.** This supplement is good for those who already have gum disease because it provides cellular energy that helps repair gum tissue. Ask your doctor what the best amount for you is—standard daily dosages range from 30 mg to 200 mg daily.

•**Magnesium.** Grinding your teeth can worsen existing gum disease (and cause all sorts of other dental problems, such as tooth decay, even if you don't have gum disease). So ask your dentist whether you should also take 50 mg to 100 mg of magnesium one hour before bedtime to relax your muscles—this helps lots of his patients who are grinders.

Best Solutions for Dry Mouth

Louis Mandel, DDS, an associate dean, a clinical professor and director of the Salivary Gland Center at Columbia University College of Dental Medicine in New York City.

Mouth dryness, known as xerostomia, is commonly thought of as a normal part of aging. But that's not true. Healthy adults continue to produce adequate amounts of saliva, but some medical conditions and certain medications can lead to dry mouth—and that can be more dangerous than you might think.

What most people don't realize: Dry mouth is more than a mere annoyance. It significantly increases risk for infection (including gum disease) and severe tooth decay. And treating the teeth does not solve the problem of dry mouth.

Low-Saliva Symptoms

Saliva is mostly water, but it also contains enzymes that break down food particles. It inhibits the growth of bacteria that can damage tooth enamel and is crucial for preventing fungal infections in the mouth. Saliva also lubricates the mouth so that we can speak and swallow.

If you don't produce enough saliva, you will, of course, notice mouth dryness. Other symptoms include cracks in the lips or the corners of the mouth, bad breath, burning of the mouth, a dry feeling in the throat and an increase in tooth decay and/or gum disease.

Self-test: You're probably producing normal amounts of saliva if you can chew a dry cracker and swallow it easily. People who consistently struggle to eat and swallow dry foods have a problem.

If you have dry mouth, your physician or dentist may want to measure your output of saliva with a Lashley cup, a device that fits over the opening of the parotid duct (the primary duct of the major salivary gland). Salivary flow is stimulated with a citric acid solution that is applied to the borders of the tongue with a cotton swab. Saliva is then collected. A healthy adult should produce between 0.5 cc and 1.2 cc of saliva (about one-tenth to one-quarter of a teaspoon) per minute per gland when stimulated.

What Causes Mouth Dryness?

Sjögren's syndrome, an autoimmune disorder, is a common cause of mouth dryness. This disease damages the glands that produce saliva and can cause swelling and pain in the joints.

Other causes of xerostomia …

•**Radiation treatments** for oral or neck cancers can permanently damage cells in the salivary glands.

Example: Radiotherapy that's used to treat oral cancer kills saliva-producing cells as the beam passes through the salivary glands.

•**Medication use.** According to the Surgeon General's report on oral health in America, more than 400 prescription and over-the-counter (OTC) drugs cause mouth dryness as a side effect.

Common offenders: Antihistamines, antidepressants, decongestants and diuretics and other blood pressure drugs.

It's rare for a single medication to cause significant dryness (though it can happen). The risk multiplies when patients are taking multiple medications that have mouth dryness as a side effect.

To find out if a medication you are taking may cause mouth dryness: Check the website for the Physicians' Desk Reference, PDRhealth.com.

•**Mouth-breathing.** Some people tend to breathe through their mouths, which can cause dryness even if they produce normal amounts of saliva. This usually occurs in those who have some kind of nasal obstruction, such as a deviated septum, or the breathing disorder sleep apnea.

To check yourself for mouth-breathing at night: Notice whether your mouth feels dry in the morning. People who mouth-breathe tend to experience the most dryness when they first wake up.

•**Dehydration.** You need adequate amounts of fluids to produce saliva. Most people get enough water from beverages and food, but older adults often forget to drink enough water. Other causes of dry mouth include uncontrolled diabetes. Frequent urination (a symptom of diabetes) may lead to dehydration and dry mouth.

Best Treatment Options

If you and your doctor determine that your mouth dryness is caused by medication, ask about switching to a drug and/or dose that doesn't have this side effect. *Also helpful…*

•**Try a saliva substitute that contains carboxymethylcellulose or hydroxyethylcellulose.** Such products, which are sold OTC at most drugstores in solutions, sprays, gels and lozenges, can be used as needed to replace moisture in the mouth. Good choices include Optimoist…Biotene Moisturizing Mouth Spray…and Entertainer's Secret.

•**Chew sugarless gum and suck on sugarless hard candies to help increase saliva flow.** Hard lemon drops are a good choice because the sourness stimulates more saliva.

•**Drink more water or suck on ice cubes to moisten your mouth and increase your fluid intake.**

•**Use a dry-mouth toothpaste such as Biotene.** It doesn't increase saliva, but it may relieve burning sensations caused by mouth dryness and is less likely to irritate dry tissues in the mouth than other toothpastes.

•**Avoid mouthwashes with alcohol.** Alcohol is a desiccant that dries tissues in the mouth. If you use a mouthwash, buy an alcohol-free version—and use it only once a day.

•**Protect your teeth with fluoride.** I advise patients who are scheduled for—or have already had—radiation treatments of the head or neck to apply fluoride gel to the teeth. Your dentist can make plastic dental trays and provide the gel. Applying fluoride for five to 10 minutes daily will help prevent tooth decay that may result from excessive mouth dryness.

CHAPTER 10

Help for Chronic Conditions

Arthritis—Easy Ways to Beat the Pain

Peter Bales, MD, a board-certified orthopedic surgeon and member of the clinical staff in the department of orthopedic surgery at the University of California at Davis Health System. A research advocate for the Arthritis Foundation (Arthritis.org), he is the author of *Osteoarthritis: Preventing and Healing Without Drugs*.

Osteoarthritis has long been considered a "wear-and-tear" disease associated with age-related changes that occur within cartilage and bone.

Now: A growing body of evidence shows that osteoarthritis may have a metabolic basis. Poor diet results in inflammatory changes and damage in cartilage cells, which in turn lead to cartilage breakdown and the development of osteoarthritis.

A recent increase in osteoarthritis cases corresponds to similar increases in diabetes and obesity, other conditions that can be fueled by poor nutrition. Dietary approaches can help prevent—or manage—all three of these conditions.

Key scientific evidence: A number of large studies, including many conducted in Europe as well as the US, suggest that a diet emphasizing plant foods and fish can support cartilage growth and impede its breakdown. People who combine an improved diet with certain supplements can reduce osteoarthritis symptoms—and possibly stop progression of the disease.

A Smarter Diet

By choosing your foods carefully, you can significantly improve the pain and stiffness caused by osteoarthritis. *How to get started...*

•**Avoid acidic foods.** The typical American diet, with its processed foods, red meat and harmful trans-fatty acids, increases acidity in the body. A high-acid environment within the joints increases free radicals, corrosive molecules that both accelerate cartilage damage and inhibit the activity of cartilage-producing cells known as chondrocytes.

A Mediterranean diet, which includes generous amounts of fruits, vegetables, whole grains, olive oil and fish, is more alkaline. (The body requires a balance of acidity and alkalinity, as measured on the pH scale.) A predominantly alkaline body chemistry inhibits free radicals and reduces inflammation.

What to do: Eat a Mediterranean-style diet, including six servings daily of vegetables…three servings of fruit…and two tablespoons of olive oil. (The acids in fruits and vegetables included in this diet are easily neutralized in the body.) Other sources of healthful fats include olives, nuts (such as walnuts), canola oil and flaxseed oil or ground flaxseed.

Important: It can take 12 weeks or more to flush out acidic toxins and reduce arthritis symptoms after switching to an alkaline diet.

•**Limit your intake of sugary and processed foods.** Most Americans consume a lot of refined carbohydrates as well as sugar-sweetened foods and soft drinks—all of which damage joints in several ways. For example, sugar causes an increase in advanced glycation endproducts (AGEs), protein molecules that bind to collagen (the connective tissue of cartilage and other tissues) and make it stiff and brittle. AGEs also appear to stimulate the production of cartilage-degrading enzymes.

What to do: Avoid processed foods, such as white flour (including cakes, cookies and crackers), white pasta and white rice, as well as soft drinks and fast food. Studies have shown that people who mainly eat foods in their whole, natural forms tend to have lower levels of AGEs and healthier cartilage.

Important: Small amounts of sugar—used to sweeten coffee or cereal, for example—will not significantly increase AGE levels.

•**Get more vitamin C.** More than 10 years ago, the Framingham study found that people who took large doses of vitamin C had a threefold reduction in the risk for osteoarthritis progression.

Vitamin C is an alkalinizing agent due to its anti-inflammatory and antioxidant properties. It blocks the inflammatory effects of free radicals. Vitamin C also decreases the formation of AGEs and reduces the chemical changes that cause cartilage breakdown.

What to do: Take a vitamin C supplement (1,000 mg daily for the prevention of osteoarthritis…2,000 mg daily if you have osteoarthritis).* Also increase your intake of vitamin C–rich foods, such as sweet red peppers, strawberries and broccoli.

•**Drink green tea.** Green tea alone won't relieve osteoarthritis pain, but people who drink green tea and switch to a healthier diet may notice an additional improvement in symptoms. That's because green tea is among the most potent sources of antioxidants, including catechins, substances that inhibit the activity of cartilage-degrading enzymes. For osteoarthritis, drink one to two cups of green tea daily. (Check with your doctor first if you take any prescription drugs.)

•**Eat fish.** Eat five to six three-ounce servings of omega-3–rich fish (such as salmon, sardines and mackerel) weekly. Omega-3s in such fish help maintain the health of joint cartilage and help curb inflammation. If you would prefer to take a fish oil supplement rather than eat fish, see the recommendation below.

Supplements That Help

Dietary changes are a first step to reducing osteoarthritis symptoms. However, the use of certain supplements also can be helpful.

•**Fish oil.** The two omega-3s in fish—docosahexaenoic acid (DHA) and eicosapentaenoic acid (EPA)—block chemical reactions in our cells that convert dietary fats into chemical messengers (such as prostaglandins), which affect the inflammatory status of our bodies. This is the same process that's inhibited by nonsteroidal anti-inflammatory drugs (NSAIDs), such as *ibuprofen* (Motrin).

What to do: If you find it difficult to eat the amount of omega-3–rich fish mentioned above, ask your doctor about taking fish oil supplements that supply a total of 1,600 mg of EPA and 800 mg of DHA daily. Look for a "pharmaceutical grade" fish oil product, such as Sealogix, available at FishOilRx. com, 888-966-3423…or RxOmega-3 Factors at iHerb.com.

If, after 12 weeks, you need more pain relief—or have a strong family history of osteoarthritis—add…

•**Glucosamine, chondroitin and MSM.** The most widely used supplements for osteoarthritis are glucosamine and chondroitin, taken singly or in combination. Most studies show that they work.

*Check with your doctor before taking any dietary supplements.

Better: A triple combination that contains methylsulfonylmethane (MSM) as well as glucosamine and chondroitin. MSM is a sulfur-containing compound that provides the raw material for cartilage regrowth. Glucosamine and chondroitin reduce osteoarthritis pain and have anti-inflammatory properties.

What to do: Take daily supplements of glucosamine (1,500 mg)...chondroitin (1,200 mg)...and MSM (1,500 mg).

Instead of—or in addition to—the fish oil and the triple combination, you may want to take...

•**SAMe.** Like MSM, S-adenosylmethionine (SAMe) is a sulfur-containing compound. It reduces the body's production of TNF-alpha, a substance that's involved in cartilage destruction. It also seems to increase cartilage production.

In one study, researchers compared SAMe to the prescription anti-inflammatory drug *celecoxib* (Celebrex). The study was double-blind (neither the patients nor the doctors knew who was getting which drug or supplement), and it continued for four months. Initially, patients taking the celecoxib reported fewer symptoms—but by the second month, there was no difference between the two groups.

Other studies have found similar results. SAMe seems to work as well as over-the-counter and/or prescription drugs for osteoarthritis, but it works more slowly. I advise patients to take it for at least three months to see effects.

What to do: Start with 200 mg of SAMe daily and increase to 400 mg daily if necessary after a few weeks.

Stay-Well Secrets for People with Diabetes or Prediabetes

Theresa Garnero, advanced practice registered nurse (APRN), certified diabetes educator (CDE) and clinical nurse manager of the Center for Diabetes Services at the California Pacific Medical Center in San Francisco. She is the author of *Your First Year with Diabetes: What to Do, Month by Month.*

Many people downplay the seriousness of diabetes. That's a mistake. Because elevated glucose can damage blood vessels, nerves, the kidneys and eyes, people with diabetes are much more likely to die from heart disease and/or kidney disease than people without diabetes—and they are at increased risk for infections, including gum disease, as well as blindness and amputation. (Nerve damage and poor circulation can allow dangerous infections to go undetected.)

And diabetes can be sneaky—increased thirst, urination and/or hunger are the most common symptoms, but many people have no symptoms and are unaware that they are sick.

Despite these sobering facts, doctors rarely have time to give their patients all the information they need to cope with the complexities of diabetes. Fortunately, diabetes educators—health-care professionals, such as registered nurses, registered dietitians and medical social workers—can give patients practical advice on the best ways to control their condition.*

Good news: Most health insurers, including Medicare, cover the cost of diabetes patients' visits with a diabetes educator.

Savvy Eating Habits

Most doctors advise people with diabetes or prediabetes to cut back on refined carbohydrates, such as cakes and cookies, and eat more fruits, vegetables and whole grains. This maximizes nutrition and promotes a healthy body weight (being overweight greatly increases diabetes risk). *Other steps to take…*

•**Drink one extra glass of water each day.** The extra fluid will help prevent dehydration, which can raise glucose levels.

•**Never skip meals—especially breakfast.** Don't assume that bypassing a meal and fasting for more than five to six hours will help lower glucose levels. It actually triggers the liver to release glucose into the bloodstream.

Better strategy: Eat three small meals daily and have snacks in between. Start with breakfast, such as a cup of low-fat yogurt and whole-wheat toast with peanut butter or a small bowl of whole-grain cereal and a handful of nuts.

Good snack options: A small apple or three graham crackers. Each of these snacks contains about 15 g of carbohydrates.

•**Practice the "plate method."** Divide a nine-inch plate in half. Fill half with vegetables, then split the other half into quarters—one for protein, such as salmon, lean meat, beans or tofu…and the other for starches, such as one-third cup of pasta or one-half cup of peas or corn. Then have a small piece of fruit. This is an easy way to practice portion control—and get the nutrients you need.

Ask yourself if you are satisfied after you take each bite. If the answer is "yes," stop eating. This simple strategy helped one of my clients lose 50 pounds.

*To find a diabetes educator near you, consult the American Association of Diabetes Educators, 800-832-6874, DiabetesEducator.org.

•**Be wary of "sugar-free" foods.** These products, including sugar-free cookies and diabetic candy, often are high in carbohydrates, which are the body's primary source of glucose. You may be better off eating the regular product, which is more satisfying. Compare the carbohydrate contents on product labels.

Get Creative with Exercise

If you have diabetes or prediabetes, you've probably been told to get more exercise. Walking is especially helpful. For those with diabetes, walking for at least two hours a week has been shown to reduce the risk for death by 30% over an eight-year period. For those with prediabetes, walking for 30 minutes five days a week reduces by about 60% the risk that your condition will progress to diabetes. *But if you'd like some other options, consider...***

•**Armchair workouts.** These exercises, which are performed while seated and are intended for people with physical limitations to standing, increase stamina, muscle tone, flexibility and coordination. For DVDs, go to Armchair Fitness.com or call 800-882-7432.

•**Strength training.** This type of exercise builds muscle, which burns more calories than fat even when you are not exercising.*** Use hand weights, exercise machines or the weight of your own body—for example, leg squats or bicep curls with no weights. Aim for two to three sessions of strength training weekly, on alternate days.

•**Stretching—even while watching TV or talking on the phone.** By building a stretching routine into your daily activities, you won't need to set aside a separate time to do it. If your body is flexible, it's easier to perform other kinds of physical activity. Stretching also promotes better circulation. Before stretching, do a brief warm-up, such as walking for five minutes and doing several arm windmills. Aim to do stretching exercises at least three times weekly, including before your other workouts.

Control Your Blood Glucose

If you are diagnosed with diabetes, blood glucose control is the immediate goal. Self-monitoring can be performed using newer devices that test blood glucose levels.

**Consult your doctor before starting a new exercise program.

***If you have high blood pressure, be sure to check with your doctor before starting a strength-training program. This type of exercise can raise blood pressure.

Good choices: LifeScan's OneTouch Ultra... Bayer's Contour...or Abbott Laboratories' FreeStyle.

The hemoglobin A1C test, which is ordered by your doctor and typically is done two to four times a year, determines how well glucose levels have been controlled over the previous two to three months.

If you have prediabetes: Don't settle for a fasting glucose test, which measures blood glucose after you have fasted overnight. It misses two-thirds of all cases of diabetes. The oral glucose tolerance test (OGTT), which involves testing glucose immediately before drinking a premixed glass of glucose and repeating the test two hours later, is more reliable. If you can't get an OGTT, ask for an A1C test and fasting glucose test.

If you have diabetes or prediabetes, you should have your blood pressure and cholesterol checked at every doctor visit and schedule regular eye exams and dental appointments. *In addition, don't overlook...*

•**Proper kidney testing.** Doctors most commonly recommend annual microalbumin and creatinine urine tests to check for kidney disease. You also may want to ask for a glomerular filtration rate test, which measures kidney function.

•**Meticulous foot care.** High glucose levels can reduce sensation in your feet, making it hard to know when you have a cut, blister or injury. In addition to seeing a podiatrist at least once a year and inspecting your own feet daily, be wary of everyday activities that can be dangerous for people with diabetes.

Stepping into hot bath water, for example, can cause a blister or skin damage that can become infected. To protect yourself, check the water temperature on your wrist or elbow before you step in. The temperature should be warm to the touch—not hot.

Stay Up to Date on Medications

Once diabetes medication has been prescribed, people with diabetes should review their drug regimen with their doctors at every visit. *Insulin is the most commonly used diabetes drug, but you may want to also ask your doctor about these relatively new medications...*

•**DPP-4 inhibitors.** These drugs include *sitagliptin* (Januvia), which lowers glucose levels by increasing the amount of insulin secreted by the pancreas. DPP-4 inhibitors are used alone or with another type of diabetes medication.

•**Symlin.** Administered with an injectable pen, *pramlintide* (Symlin) helps control blood glucose and reduces appetite, which may help with weight loss. It is used in addition to insulin.

If you have prediabetes or diabetes: Always consult a pharmacist or doctor before taking any over-the-counter products. Cold medicines with a high sugar content may raise your blood glucose, for example, and wart removal products may cause skin ulcers. Pay close attention to drug label warnings.

Supplements That Help Manage Diabetes

Mark A. Stengler, NMD, licensed naturopathic medical doctor in private practice, Stengler Center for Integrative Medicine, Encinitas, California...author of many books, including *The Natural Physician's Healing Therapies* and coauthor of *Prescription for Natural Cures.*

L ifestyle change has always been the cornerstone treatment for people with type 2 diabetes. Beyond that, natural approaches are rarely discussed. I recommend a number of plant-based remedies for those with diabetes, some of which date back hundreds, even thousands, of years...

Type 2 diabetes absolutely can be prevented and, in certain cases, even reversed with diet, exercise and appropriate dietary supplements. The following are some of my own "best practice" advice for prevention, maintenance and symptom management of this lifestyle-related disease.

To prevent diabetes...

•**Curb sugar cravings with *gymnema sylvestre*.** A staple of Ayurvedic medicine, this herb helps curb cravings for sugary foods that throw your blood glucose levels off balance. Scientists speculate that it works by positively influencing insulin-producing cells in the pancreas.

Gymnema sylvestre works best when used in combination with other glucose-balancing herbs, such as bitter melon and fenugreek. Ask your doctor for advice on the best combination and dosage for you.

•**Chromium can normalize sugar levels.** Your body requires adequate levels of chromium to properly control blood glucose levels. This essential trace mineral aids in the uptake of blood sugar into the body's cells, where it can be used to generate energy more efficiently. It's also helpful in reducing sweet cravings.

I advise up to 1,000 micrograms of chromium a day (under your physician's supervision). This is a good mineral to take with gymnema.

•**Regulate blood sugar with fiber and fiber supplements.** Soluble fiber helps prevent or control prediabetes and diabetes by slowing the rate at which intestines release glucose into the bloodstream, thus modulating fluctuations in blood sugar levels. Rich sources of soluble fiber include plant foods, such as legumes, oat bran, rye, barley, broccoli, carrots, artichokes, peas, prunes, berries and bananas. In a small study in Taiwan, scientists found that supplementation with glucomannan (a soluble dietary fiber made from konjac flour) lowered elevated levels of blood lipids, cholesterol and glucose in people with diabetes.

Most Americans eat too much junk food and too little fiber. For my patients who fall into that category, I typically prescribe one glucomannan capsule 30 minutes before lunch and dinner, and another before bedtime with a large glass of water.

Managing symptoms and minimizing complications...

•**Boost antioxidant levels with alpha-lipoic acid.** This powerful antioxidant kills free radicals that damage cells and cause pain, inflammation, burning, tingling and numbness in people who have peripheral neuropathy (nerve damage) caused by diabetes. Studies also suggest that alpha-lipoic acid (ALA) enables the body to utilize glucose more efficiently.

Alpha-lipoic acid can be taken daily under a physician's supervision.

•**Decrease blood glucose levels with chamomile tea.** Drinking chamomile tea, a rich source of antioxidants, may help prevent diabetes complications, such as blindness, nerve damage and kidney problems, according to recent research by UK and Japanese scientists.

Drink chamomile tea along with antioxidant-rich black, white and green teas.

•**Take omega-3 fatty acids to reduce inflammation.** These healthy fats improve the body's ability to respond to insulin, reduce inflammation, lower blood lipids and prevent excessive blood clotting. Good dietary sources of omega-3 fatty acids include cold-water fish, such as salmon or cod (eat two or three times a week), olive or canola oil, flaxseed and English walnuts.

My advice: Unless you know you are getting sufficient omega-3 fatty acids in your diet, it's good to take a daily fish oil supplement that contains about

1,000 mg of the omega-3 fatty acid *eicosapentaenoic acid* (EPA) and about 500 mg of the omega-3 fatty acid *docosahexaenoic acid* (DHA).

Caution: Because many dietary supplements lower blood sugar, and fish oil supplements may alter the way anticoagulant therapy functions, it is critical to work closely with your doctor before and while taking any of the above supplements. He/she will prescribe the right doses for you and also may suggest that you alter other medications accordingly.

Don't Neglect the ABCs of Diabetes Self-Care

When addressing a difficult disease such as diabetes, all the nutrients and vitamins in the world will do no good if you do not also follow the basics of diabetes self-care. Maintain a healthy weight…get 20 to 30 minutes of exercise most days of the week…follow a diet that emphasizes lean proteins and healthy fats and limits simple carbohydrates…monitor blood glucose levels…and take diabetes, blood pressure and cholesterol medicine as prescribed by your physician. Even as simple a measure as taking a 10-minute walk after each meal can keep blood sugar under control. Start today.

The Diabetes Complication That Kills More People Than Most Cancers

James M. Horton, MD, chair of the Standards and Practice Guidelines Committee of the Infectious Diseases Society of America, IDSociety.org. Dr. Horton is also chief of the department of infectious disease and attending faculty physician in the department of internal medicine, both at Carolinas Medical Center in Charlotte, North Carolina.

A foot or leg amputation is one of the most dreaded complications of diabetes. In the US, more than 65,000 such amputations occur each year.

But the tragedy does not stop there. According to recent research, about half of all people who have a foot amputation die within five years of the surgery—a worse mortality rate than most cancers. That's partly because people with diabetes who have amputations often have poorer glycemic control and more complications such as kidney disease. Amputation also can lead to increased pressure on the remaining limb and the possibility of new ulcers and infections.

Latest development: To combat the increasingly widespread problem of foot infections and amputations, new guidelines for the diagnosis and treatment of diabetic foot infections have been created by the Infectious Diseases Society of America (IDSA).

What you need to know…

How Foot Infections Start

Diabetes can lead to foot infections in two main ways—peripheral neuropathy (nerve damage that can cause loss of sensation in the feet)…and ischemia (inadequate blood flow).

To understand why these conditions can be so dangerous, think back to the last time you had a pebble inside your shoe. How long did it take before the irritation became unbearable? Individuals with peripheral neuropathy and ischemia usually don't feel any pain in their feet. Without pain, the pebble will stay in the shoe and eventually cause a sore on the sole of the foot.

Similarly, people with diabetes will not feel the rub of an ill-fitting shoe or the pressure of standing on one foot too long, so they are at risk of developing pressure sores or blisters.

These small wounds can lead to big trouble. About 25% of people with diabetes will develop a foot ulcer—ranging from mild to severe—at some point in their lives. Any ulcer, blister, cut or irritation has the potential to become infected. If the infection becomes too severe to treat effectively with antibiotics, amputation of a foot or leg may be the only way to prevent the infection from spreading throughout the body and save the person's life.

A Fast-Moving Danger

Sores on the foot can progress rapidly. While some foot sores remain unchanged for months, it is possible for an irritation to lead to an open wound (ulcer), infection and amputation in as little as a few days. That is why experts recommend that people with diabetes seek medical care promptly for any open sore on the feet or any new area of redness or irritation that could possibly lead to an open wound.

Important: Fully half of diabetic foot ulcers are infected and require immediate medical treatment and sometimes hospitalization.

Don't try to diagnose yourself—diagnosis requires a trained medical expert. An ulcer that appears very small on the surface could have actually spread underneath the skin, so you very well could be seeing just a small portion of the infection.

What Your Doctor Will Do

The first step is to identify the bacteria causing the infection. To do this, physicians collect specimens from deep inside the wound. Once the bacteria have been identified, the proper antibiotics can be prescribed.

Physicians also need to know the magnitude of the infection—for example, whether there is bone infection, abscesses or other internal problems. Therefore, all diabetes patients who have new foot infections should have X-rays. If more detailed imaging is needed, an MRI or a bone scan may be ordered.

The doctor will then classify the wound and infection as mild, moderate or severe and create a treatment plan.

How to Get the Best Treatment

Each person's wound is unique, so there are no cookie-cutter treatment plans. *However, most treatment plans should include...*

•**A diabetes foot-care team.** For moderate or severe infections, a team of experts should coordinate treatment. This will be done for you—by the hospital or your primary care physician. The number of specialists on the team depends on the patient's specific needs but may include experts in podiatry and vascular surgery. In rural or smaller communities, this may be done via online communication with experts from larger hospitals (telemedicine).

•**Antibiotic treatment.** Milder infections usually involve a single bacterium. Antibiotics will typically be needed for about one week. With more severe infections, multiple bacteria are likely involved, so you will require multiple antibiotics, and treatment will need to continue for a longer period—sometimes four weeks or more if bone is affected.

If the infection is severe...or even moderate but complicated by, say, poor blood circulation, hospitalization may be required for a few days to a few weeks, depending on the course of the recovery.

•**Wound care.** Many patients who have foot infections receive antibiotic therapy only, which is often insufficient. Proper wound care is also necessary. In addition to frequent wound cleansing and dressing changes, this may include surgical removal of dead tissue (debridement)...and the use of specially designed shoes or shoe inserts—provided by a podiatrist—to redistribute pressure off the wound (off-loading).

•**Surgery.** Surgery doesn't always mean amputation. It is sometimes used not only to remove dead or damaged tissue or bone but also to improve blood flow to the foot.

If an infection fails to improve: The first question physicians know to ask is: "Is the patient complying with wound care instructions?" Too many patients lose a leg because they don't take their antibiotics as prescribed or care for the injury as prescribed.

Never forget: Following your doctors' specific orders could literally mean the difference between having one leg or two.

Foot Care Is Critical If You Have Diabetes

To protect yourself from foot injuries…

•**Never walk barefoot, even around the house.**

•**Don't wear sandals**—the straps can irritate the side of the foot.

•**Wear thick socks with soft leather shoes.** Leather is a good choice because it "breathes," molds to the feet and does not retain moisture. Laced-up shoes with cushioned soles provide the most support.

In addition, pharmacies carry special "diabetic socks" that protect and cushion your feet without cutting off circulation at the ankle. These socks usually have no seams that could chafe. They also wick moisture away from feet, which reduces risk for infection and foot ulcers.

•**See a podiatrist.** This physician can advise you on the proper care of common foot problems, such as blisters, corns and ingrown toenails. A podiatrist can also help you find appropriate footwear—even if you have foot deformities.

Ask your primary care physician or endocrinologist for a recommendation, or consult the American Podiatric Medical Association, APMA.org.

Also: Inspect your feet every day. Otherwise, you may miss a developing infection. Look for areas of redness, blisters or open sores, particularly in the areas most prone to injury—the bottoms and bony inner and outer edges of the feet.

If you see any sign of a sore, seek prompt medical care. You should also see a doctor if you experience an infected or ingrown toenail, callus formation, bunions or other deformity, fissured (cracked) skin on your feet or you notice any change in sensation.

Natural Ways to Quiet Tremors

Monique Giroux, MD, a neurologist and medical director and cofounder of the Movement & Neuroperformance Center of Colorado in Englewood, Centerfor Movement.org. She is the author of *Optimizing Health with Parkinson's Disease.*

Most people think of tremors—rhythmic trembling in your hands, voice, head or other parts of your body—as a red flag for neurological disorders such as Parkinson's disease and multiple sclerosis (MS).

That can be true. But this constant shakiness can also accompany a wide range of other conditions, including so-called essential tremor (ET), a chronic but harmless disorder that often is inherited and affects an estimated seven million Americans—a greater number than those affected by MS and Parkinson's disease. In some people, tremors also can occur as a side effect of common prescription drugs such as certain antidepressants, asthma inhalers, seizure medicines and immune-suppressing drugs. Even pain and anxiety can cause mild shaking or worsen tremors that are due to disease or medication.

If you suffer from tremors, there's no question how disruptive the problem can be to everyday life. Simple movements most of us take for granted—such as shaving, eating or simply writing a check—can turn into a shaky endurance test.

But quieting tremors is no small feat. Medications such as antiseizure drugs and mild tranquilizers are effective only about half of the time and can have troubling side effects, including drowsiness and confusion. Injections of botulinum toxin (Botox) can help head and voice tremors but are less effective for hand tremors because weakness can result as a side effect. An invasive procedure called deep brain stimulation (DBS) is reserved for the worst cases. This treatment, which can be quite effective, involves surgically implanting electrodes in the brain that are connected to a pacemaker placed under the skin near the collarbone. Electrical pulses are continuously delivered to block the impulses that cause tremors.

Good news: If drugs or surgery aren't for you or leave you with lingering symptoms, several natural therapies can help calm tremors by easing the stress and altering the brain chemicals and emotional responses that exacerbate the condition.

Important: Before trying natural remedies, be sure to avoid caffeine, smoking and/or excess alcohol—all of which can worsen tremors. Also, make regular exercise (especially strength training) a priority—tremors are more common when muscles become fatigued. *Natural treatments to tame any type of tremor…**

Aromatherapy

Breathing in the aroma of certain flowers and herbs can reduce tremors by enhancing brain levels of gamma-aminobutyric acid (GABA), a widely circulated neurotransmitter with proven stress-fighting effects. Raising GABA levels helps calm the overexcited neurons that can worsen tremors. *What to try for tremors…*

•**Lavender.** This fragrant blue-violet flower has been shown in a number of small studies to produce calming, soothing and sedative effects when its scent is inhaled. Lavender essential oil is widely available and can be inhaled in the bath (add five to eight drops to bath water for a long soak) or by dabbing a drop on your neck or temples.

Supplements

Certain supplements can ease tremors by enhancing muscle relaxation and/ or reducing the body's overall stress levels or load of inflammatory chemicals, which can play a role in tremors caused by neurodegenerative diseases. Check with your doctor to make sure these supplements don't interact with any medication you may be taking and won't affect any chronic condition you may have…**

•**Magnesium.** This mineral helps to regulate nerve impulses and muscle contraction. Magnesium-rich foods include sesame seeds, beans, nuts, avocados and leafy greens. To ensure that you're getting enough magnesium, consider taking a supplement.

Typical dose to ease tremors: 200 mg to 400 mg daily.

•**Fish oil.** The omega-3 fatty acids in fish oil offer proven anti-inflammatory effects—systemic inflammation is implicated in neurodegenerative diseases such as MS and Parkinson's disease. Fish oil is abundant in fatty fish such as salmon, albacore tuna, mackerel and herring. Aim for two servings per week. If you don't like fish, consider trying a supplement.

Typical dose to ease tremors: 1,000 mg to 1,500 mg daily.

*Consult your doctor before trying the diet and/or supplements described here—especially if you take any medication or have kidney or liver disease.

**Because supplements aren't regulated by the FDA for purity, I advise looking for products that bear the "USP-verified" stamp on the label—this means they have met rigorous testing standards to ensure quality by the scientific nonprofit US Pharmacopeial Convention.

•**Valerian, skullcap and passionflower.** These calming herbs have been successfully used as part of a regimen to ease tremors. The supplements can be found in combination products, including capsules, teas and tinctures. Follow instructions on the label.

Beat Tremors with Your Mind

If you suffer from tremors, it's common to think—Oh no...my arm (or other body part) is shaking again...this is so embarrassing! I hate this! While such thoughts are perfectly natural when tremors emerge, they are potentially destructive when trying to calm your condition.

What helps: Mindfulness can reset this negative thought pattern so that you stop viewing tremors as a problem, which only leads to distress that often worsens the condition.

Mindfulness is more than just relaxation. Often done in conjunction with deep-breathing exercises, mindfulness helps you simply observe your thoughts, feelings and sensations and let them pass without judging them, labeling them or trying to control them. By reducing the distress you feel about the tremors, you are no longer fueling the condition.

You can learn mindfulness from CDs or books. My recommendations: Consult your local hospital to see if it offers mindfulness-based stress-reduction classes. Also consider trying other mind-body therapies that may help, such as hypnosis, biofeedback and breath work.

Best Nondrug Approaches for Parkinson's

Michael S. Okun, MD, professor and chair of the department of neurology and co-director of the Center for Movement Disorders and Neurorestoration at the University of Florida College of Medicine in Gainesville. He is also the medical director at the National Parkinson Foundation and has written more than 400 medical journal articles. Dr. Okun's latest book is *10 Breakthrough Therapies for Parkinson's Disease.*

The telltale tremors, muscle stiffness and other movement problems that plague people with Parkinson's disease make even the mundane activities of daily living—such as brushing teeth, cooking and dressing—more difficult.

What's new: Even though medication—such as levodopa (L-dopa) and newer drugs including pramipexole and selegiline—have long been the main treatment to control Parkinson's symptoms, researchers are discovering more and more nondrug therapies that can help.

Among the best nondrug approaches (each can be used with Parkinson's medication)...

Exercise

For people with Parkinson's, exercise is like a drug. It raises neurotrophic factors, proteins that promote the growth and health of neurons. Research consistently shows that exercise can improve motor symptoms (such as walking speed and stability) and quality of life.

For the best results: Exercise 30 to 60 minutes every single day. Aim to work hard enough to break a sweat, but back off if you get too fatigued—especially the following day (this indicates the body is not recovering properly). Parkinson's symptoms can worsen with over-exercise. *Smart exercise habits...*

For better gait speed: Choose a lower-intensity exercise, such as walking on a treadmill (but hold on to the balance bars), rather than high-intensity exercise (such as running), which has a higher risk for falls and other injuries.

A recent study showed that a walking group of Parkinson's patients performed better than a group of patients who ran.

Important safety tip: Parkinson's patients should exercise with a partner and take precautions to prevent falls—for example, minimizing distractions, such as ringing cell phones.

For aerobic exercise: Use a recumbent bicycle or rowing machine and other exercises that don't rely on balance.

For strength and flexibility: Do stretching and progressive resistance training.

Excellent resource: For a wide variety of exercises, including aerobic workouts, standing and sitting stretches, strengthening moves, balance exercises and fall-prevention tips, the National Parkinson Foundation's *Fitness Counts* book is available as a free download at Parkinson.org/pd-library/books/fitness-counts.

For balance: Researchers are now discovering that yoga postures, tai chi (with its slow, controlled movements) and certain types of dancing (such as the tango, which involves rhythmic forward-and-backward steps) are excellent ways to improve balance.

Coffee and Tea

Could drinking coffee or tea help with Parkinson's? According to research, it can—when consumed in the correct amounts.

Here's why: Caffeine blocks certain receptors in the brain that regulate the neurotransmitter dopamine, which becomes depleted and leads to the impaired motor coordination that characterizes Parkinson's. In carefully controlled studies, Parkinson's patients who ingested low doses of caffeine—about 100 mg twice daily—had improved motor symptoms, such as tremors and stiffness, compared with people who had no caffeine or higher doses of caffeine.

My advice: Have 100 mg of caffeine (about the amount in one six-ounce cup of home-brewed coffee or two cups of black or green tea) twice a day—once in the morning and once in the mid-afternoon.

Note: Even decaffeinated coffee has about 10 mg to 25 mg of caffeine per cup.

Supplements

Researchers have studied various supplements for years to identify ones that could help manage Parkinson's symptoms and/or boost the effects of levodopa, but large studies have failed to prove that these supplements provide such benefits.

However, because Parkinson's is a complex disease that can cause about 20 different motor and nonmotor symptoms that evolve over time, the existing research may not apply to everyone. *Some people with Parkinson's may benefit from…*

•**Coenzyme Q10 (CoQ10).** This supplement promotes the health of the body's mitochondria ("energy generators" in the cells), which are believed to play a role in Parkinson's. In a large study, people with Parkinson's who took 1,200 mg per day showed some improvement in symptoms over a 16-month study period. However, follow-up studies found no beneficial effects.

•**Riboflavin and alpha-lipoic acid** are among the other supplements that are continuing to be studied.

Important: If you wish to try these or other supplements, be sure to consult your doctor to ensure that there are no possible interactions with your other medications.

Marijuana

A few small studies have concluded that marijuana can improve some neurological symptoms, but larger studies are needed to show benefits for Parkinson's patients, especially for symptoms such as depression and anxiety.

However: Marijuana is challenging for several reasons—first, it is illegal in most states. If you do live in a state that allows medical marijuana use, it has possible side effects—for example, it can impair balance and driving...it is difficult to know the exact dosage, even if it's purchased from a dispensary... and with marijuana edibles (such as cookies and candies), the effects may take longer to appear, and you may accidentally ingest too much.

If you want to try marijuana: Work closely with your doctor to help you avoid such pitfalls.

Seeing the Right Doctor

For anyone with Parkinson's, it's crucial to see a neurologist and, if possible, one who has advanced training in Parkinson's disease and movement disorders.

Important new finding: A large study showed that patients treated by a neurologist had a lower risk for hip fracture and were less likely to be placed in a nursing facility. They were also 22% less likely to die during the four-year study.

Simple Stretches That Really Do Relieve Pain

Ben Benjamin, PhD, a sports medicine and muscular therapy practitioner since 1963. He is the author of several books, including *Listen to Your Pain: The Active Person's Guide to Understanding, Identifying, and Treating Pain and Injury.* BenBenjamin.com

If you suffer from pain or stiffness due to an injury, arthritis or even a neurological disorder, such as Parkinson's disease or multiple sclerosis, a type of bodywork known as Active Isolated Stretching (AIS) may give you more relief than you ever thought possible.

What makes AIS different: While most other stretching techniques recommend doing each stretch for 30 seconds or longer, AIS uses brief, two-second stretches that are done eight to 10 times each.

What's the advantage of quick, repeated stretches? This approach gives the muscle a full stretch without triggering its stretch reflex—an automatic defense mechanism that causes the muscle to contract and ultimately undo many of the stretch's benefits. The result is that muscles stretch more efficiently and avoid the buildup of waste products that lead to muscle soreness.

Developed by American kinesiologist Aaron Mattes about 35 years ago, AIS also stretches each muscle group at a variety of different angles, thus stretching all muscle fibers equally.

A Mini Regimen

To get a sense of AIS, try the stretches in this article. While doing each one, slowly count to yourself "one-one thousand, two-one thousand"—never any longer than two seconds. Always exhale while performing the stretch and inhale as you return to the starting position.

The first repetition of each stretch should be gentle…the second should go up to the point where you begin to feel resistance. Subsequent repetitions should push just beyond this point (with the help of your hands, a rope or other aid, if necessary) to go a few degrees further each time, thus providing a maximum stretch. If you feel discomfort during a stretch, stop the stretch at that point. If a stretch feels painful from the start, then skip it.

Daily AIS exercises that help relieve common types of pain…*

Shoulder Stretches

Purpose: To help prevent muscle strain and joint sprain by increasing flexibility.

1. With your right elbow bent, position your right arm at a 90° angle in front of your body. Place your right palm on the back of your right shoulder. Exhale and extend your flexed arm upward as far as possible. Gently assist the stretch with your left hand. Repeat eight to 10 times on each side.

2. With your right elbow bent and your right arm positioned at a 90° angle in front of your body, place your right palm on the back of your right shoulder. Drop a two- to three-foot rope over your right shoulder and grasp the bottom of it with your left hand. Gently pull the rope to move your right arm upward behind your neck at a 45° angle for a maximum stretch. Return to the starting position after each repetition. Repeat eight to 10 times on each side.

*Check with your doctor before performing these movements.

Neck Stretches

Purpose: To help prevent neck injuries, relieve stiffness and improve range of motion.

1. Tuck your chin as close to your neck as possible. Put both your hands on the back of your head and, while keeping your back straight, gently bend your neck forward, bringing your chin as close to your chest as you can. Return to starting position. Repeat 10 times.

2. Gently bend your head to the right side, moving your right ear as close as possible to the top of your right shoulder. Exhale and place your right hand on the left side of your head to gently extend the stretch. Keep your left shoulder down. Focus your eyes on a point directly in front of your body to keep your head in an aligned position. Repeat 10 times on both sides.

Getting Started

For people who are new to AIS, I advise working with an AIS practitioner for hands-on instruction. If the movements are done incorrectly, you will get no benefits and could even hurt yourself. To find a practitioner near you, go to StretchingUSA.com and click on the "Practitioner Directory" link. Sessions are not typically covered by insurance and usually range from $50 to $150 per session. The website also offers books, including *Specific Stretching for Everyone*, and DVDs if you prefer to learn a complete AIS regimen on your own.

Four Secrets to Easier Breathing... Simple Ways to Help Yourself

Gerard J. Criner, MD, a professor of medicine and director of pulmonary and critical care medicine at Temple Lung Center at Temple University School of Medicine in Philadelphia. He is codirector of the Center for Inflammation, Translational and Clinical Lung Research.

I f you can't catch your breath, walking, climbing stairs or simply carrying on a conversation can be a challenge.

When breathing is a struggle, you wouldn't think that exercise is the answer. But it can be a solution for people with chronic obstructive pulmonary disease (COPD) or heart failure or even for healthy people who occasionally become short of breath.*

Four better-breathing techniques that really help...

Pursed-Lip Breathing

When you're feeling short of breath, inhale through your nose for two seconds, then pucker your lips as if you were going to whistle or blow out a candle. Exhale through pursed lips for four seconds.

How it helps: It prolongs the respiratory cycle and gives you more time to empty your lungs. This is particularly important if you have emphysema. With emphysema, air gets trapped in the lungs. The trapped air causes the lungs to overinflate, which reduces the amount of force that they're able to generate. This results in a buildup of carbon dioxide that makes it difficult to breathe.

You may need to do this only when you're more active than usual and short of breath. Or you may breathe better when you do it often.

Changing Positions

Simply changing how you stand or sit can improve breathing when you're feeling winded.

How it helps: Certain positions (see below) help muscles around the diaphragm work more efficiently to promote easier breathing.

Examples: While sitting, lean your chest forward...rest your elbows on your knees...and relax your upper-body muscles. When standing, bend forward at the waist and rest your hands on a table or the back of a chair. Or back up to a wall...support yourself with your hips...and lean forward and put your hands on your thighs.

Controlled Coughing

Your lungs produce excessive mucus when you have COPD. The congestion makes it harder to breathe. It also increases the risk for pneumonia and other lung infections. A normal, explosive cough is not effective at removing mucus. In fact, out-of-control coughing can cause airways to collapse and trap even

---

*If you don't have COPD, you should see a doctor if you have shortness of breath after only slight activity or while resting, or if shortness of breath wakes you up at night or requires you to sleep propped up to breathe.

more mucus. A controlled cough is more effective (and requires less oxygen and energy). You also can use this technique to help clear mucus from the lungs when you have a cold.

How to do it: Sit on a chair or the edge of your bed with both feet on the floor. Fold your arms around your midsection...breathe in slowly through your nose...then lean forward while pressing your arms against your abdomen. Lightly cough two or three times. Repeat as needed.

Important: Taking slow, gentle breaths through your nose while using this technique will prevent mucus from moving back into the airways.

Cold-Air Assistance

This is a quick way to breathe better. When you are short of breath—or doing an activity that you know will lead to breathlessness, such as walking on a treadmill—position a fan so that it blows cool air on your face. You also can splash your face with cold water if you become short of breath.

How it helps: Cool air and water stimulate the trigeminal nerve in the face, which slows respiration and helps ease shortness of breath. That's why the treadmills and exercise bikes used in respiratory-rehabilitation facilities are often equipped with small fans.

When to Get Breathing Help from a Professional

You can do many breathing exercises on your own without the help of a health professional. For the techniques below, however, it's best to first consult a respiratory therapist (ask your doctor for a referral) to ensure that you know how to do the exercise properly. You can then continue on your own.

•**Paced breathing for endurance.** This technique is useful for people who have COPD and/or heart failure, since it improves lung capacity and heart function.

How it helps: With practice, this technique can increase your cardio-respiratory endurance by 30% to 40%. To perform the exercise, a metronome is set at a rate that's faster than your usual respiratory rate. Your therapist will encourage you to breathe as hard and as fast as you can for, say, about 15 minutes. (Beginners might do it for only a few minutes at a time.)

Example: The metronome may be set for 20 breaths per minute to start, and you may eventually work up to 40 breaths per minute.

You'll notice that breathing becomes easier when you're doing various activities—for instance, when you're exercising, climbing stairs or taking brisk walks.

•**Inspiratory muscle training.** Think of this as a workout for your breathing muscles. It is especially helpful for people with COPD or other lung diseases and those recovering from respiratory failure. People who strengthen these muscles can improve their breathing efficiency by 25% to 30%.

How it helps: For this breathing exercise, you'll use a device known as an inspiratory muscle trainer, which includes a mouthpiece, a one-way valve and resistance settings. When you inhale, the one-way valve closes. You're forced to use effort to breathe against resistance. Then, the valve opens so that you can exhale normally. This breathing exercise is typically performed for 15 minutes twice a day. You can buy these devices online.

Good choice: The Threshold Inspiratory Muscle Trainer, available at Fitnes Smart.com for $59.95.

CHAPTER 11

Brain and Memory Health

An Alzheimer's Prevention Plan Made Simple

Kenneth S. Kosik, MD, the Harriman Professor of Neuroscience Research and codirector of the Neuroscience Research Institute at the University of California, Santa Barbara, where he specializes in the causes and treatments of neurodegeneration, particularly Alzheimer's disease. Dr. Kosik is coauthor of *Outsmarting Alzheimer's*.

I f someone told you that there was a pill with no side effects and strong evidence showing that it helps prevent Alzheimer's disease, would you take it? Of course, you would!

The truth is, there's no such "magic bullet," but most adults do have the ability to dramatically decrease their risk for this dreaded disease.

A window of opportunity: According to the latest scientific evidence, slowing or blocking Alzheimer's plaques (buildups of dangerous protein fragments), which are now known to develop years before memory loss and other symptoms are noticeable, could be the key to stopping this disease.

As a neuroscientist who has researched Alzheimer's for 25 years, I try to incorporate healthful practices into my own daily routine to help prevent Alzheimer's. *Here are life-changing steps to follow…*

STEP 1: **Make exercise exciting.** You may know that frequent exercise—particularly aerobic exercise, which promotes blood flow to the brain—is the most effective Alzheimer's prevention strategy. Unfortunately, many people become bored and stop exercising.

Scientific evidence: Because exercise raises levels of brain-derived neurotrophic factor, it promotes the growth of new brain cells and may help prevent shrinkage of the hippocampus (a part of the brain involved in memory).

What I do: Most days, I spend 35 minutes on an elliptical trainer, followed by some weight training (increasing muscle mass helps prevent diabetes—an Alzheimer's risk factor). To break up the monotony, I go mountain biking on sunny days. I advise patients who have trouble sticking to an exercise regimen to try out the new virtual-reality equipment available in many gyms. While riding a stationary bike, for example, you can watch a monitor that puts you in the Tour de France!

Also helpful: To keep your exercise regimen exciting, go dancing. A recent 20-year study found that dancing reduced dementia risk more than any other type of exercise—perhaps because many types of dancing (such as tango, salsa and Zumba) involve learning new steps and aerobic activity. Do the type of dancing that appeals to you most.

STEP 2: **Keep your eating plan simple.** A nutritious diet is important for Alzheimer's prevention, but many people assume that they'll have to make massive changes, so they get overwhelmed and don't even try. To avoid this trap, keep it simple—all healthful diets have a few common elements, including an emphasis on antioxidant-rich foods (such as fruit and vegetables)…not too much red meat…and a limited amount of processed foods that are high in sugar, fat or additives.

Scientific evidence: Research has shown that people who consume more than four daily servings of vegetables have a 40% lower rate of cognitive decline than those who get less than one daily serving.

What I do: I try to eat more vegetables, particularly broccoli, cauliflower and other crucifers—there's strong evidence of their brain-protective effects.

Helpful: I'm not a veggie lover, so I roast vegetables with olive oil in the oven to make them more appetizing. Whenever possible, I use brain-healthy spices such as rosemary and turmeric.

STEP 3: **Guard your sleep.** During the day, harmful waste products accumulate in the brain. These wastes, including the amyloid protein that's linked to Alzheimer's, are mainly eliminated at night during deep (stages 3 and 4) sleep.

Scientific evidence: In a long-term Swedish study, men who reported poor sleep were 1.5 times more likely to develop Alzheimer's than those with better sleep.

Regardless of your age, you need a good night's sleep. While ideal sleep times vary depending on the person, sleeping less than six hours or more than nine hours nightly is linked to increased risk for cardiovascular disease—another Alzheimer's risk factor. If you don't feel rested when you wake up, talk to your doctor about your sleep quality.

What I do: I often take a 10-minute nap during the day. Brief naps (especially between 2 pm and 4 pm, which syncs with most people's circadian rhythms) can be restorative.

STEP 4: **Don't be a loner.** Having regular social interaction is strongly associated with healthy aging.

Scientific evidence: Older adults who frequently spend time with others—for example, sharing meals and volunteering—have about a 70% lower rate of cognitive decline than those who don't socialize much.

What I do: To stay socially active, I regularly Skype, attend conferences and stay in touch with other scientists and postdoc students.

If you're lonely, any form of social interaction is better than none. One study found that people who used computers regularly—to write e-mails, for example—were less lonely than those who didn't. If you can't connect in person, do a video chat or Facebook update at least once a day.

Also helpful: Having a pet. Pets are sometimes better listeners than spouses!

STEP 5: **Stay calm.** People who are often stressed are more likely to experience brain shrinkage.

Scientific evidence: In a three-year study of people with mild cognitive impairment (a condition that often precedes Alzheimer's), those with severe anxiety had a 135% increased risk for Alzheimer's, compared with those who were calmer.

What I do: I go for long walks.

Other great stress reducers: Having a positive mental attitude, deep breathing, yoga, tai chi, meditation—and even watching funny movies. Practice what works for you.

STEP 6: **Push yourself intellectually.** So-called "brain workouts" help prevent Alzheimer's—perhaps by increasing cognitive reserve (the stored memories/cognitive skills that you can draw on later in life)...and possibly by accelerating the growth of new brain cells.

Scientific evidence: In an important study, older adults (including those with a genetic risk factor for Alzheimer's) who frequently read, played board games or engaged in other mental activities were able to postpone the development of the disease by almost a decade.

But don't fool yourself—if you're an accomplished pianist, then banging out a tune won't help much even though a nonmusician is likely to benefit from learning to play. Push your mental abilities—do math problems in your head, memorize a poem, become a tutor, etc.

What I do: To challenge myself intellectually, I read novels and practice my foreign language skills—I do research in Latin America, so I work on my Spanish.

Five Surprising Ways to Prevent Alzheimer's: #1: Check Your Tap Water

Marwan Sabbagh, MD, director of Banner Sun Health Research Institute, Sun City, Arizona. He is author of *The Alzheimer's Prevention Cookbook: 100 Recipes to Boost Brain Health.* MarwanSabbaghMD.com

Every 68 seconds, another American develops Alzheimer's disease, the fatal brain disease that steals memory and personality. It's the fifth-leading cause of death among people age 65 and older.

You can lower your likelihood of getting Alzheimer's disease by reducing controllable and well-known risk factors (see end of article). *But new scientific research reveals that there are also little-known "secret" risk factors that you can address...*

1. Copper in Tap Water

A scientific paper published in *Journal of Trace Elements in Medicine and Biology* theorizes that inorganic copper found in nutritional supplements and in drinking water is an important factor in today's Alzheimer's epidemic.

Science has established that amyloid-beta plaques—inflammation-causing cellular debris found in the brains of people with Alzheimer's—contain high levels of copper. Animal research shows that small amounts of inorganic copper in drinking water worsen Alzheimer's. Studies on people have linked the combination of copper and a high-fat diet to memory loss and mental decline. It may be that copper sparks amyloid-beta plaques to generate more oxidation and inflammation, further injuring brain cells.

What to do: There is plenty of copper in our diets—no one needs additional copper from a multivitamin/mineral supplement. Look for a supplement with no copper or a minimal amount (500 micrograms).

I also recommend filtering water. Water-filter pitchers, such as ones by Brita, can reduce the presence of copper. I installed a reverse-osmosis water filter in my home a few years ago when the evidence for the role of copper in Alzheimer's became compelling.

2. Vitamin D Deficiency

Mounting evidence shows that a low blood level of vitamin D may increase Alzheimer's risk.

A 2013 study in *Journal of Alzheimer's Disease* analyzed 10 studies exploring the link between vitamin D and Alzheimer's. Researchers found that low blood levels of vitamin D were linked to a 40% increased risk for Alzheimer's.

The researchers from UCLA, also writing in *Journal of Alzheimer's Disease*, theorize that vitamin D may protect the brain by reducing amyloid-beta and inflammation.

What to do: The best way to make sure that your blood level of vitamin D is protective is to ask your doctor to test it—and then, if needed, to help you correct your level to greater than 60 nanograms per milliliter (ng/mL). That correction may require 1,000 IU to 2,000 IU of vitamin D daily…or another individualized supplementation strategy.

Important: When your level is tested, make sure that your doctor uses the 25-hydroxyvitamin D, or 25(OH)D, test and not the 1.25-dihydroxyvitamin D test. The latter test does not accurately measure blood levels of vitamin D but is sometimes incorrectly ordered. Also, ask for your exact numerical results. Levels above 30 ng/mL are considered "normal," but in my view, the 60 ng/mL level is the minimum that is protective.

3. Hormone-Replacement Therapy After Menopause

Research shows that starting hormone-replacement therapy (HRT) within five years of entering menopause and using hormones for 10 or more years reduces the risk for Alzheimer's by 30%. But a new 11-year study of 1,768 women, published in *Neurology*, shows that those who started a combination of estrogen-progestin therapy five years or more after the onset of menopause had a 93% higher risk for Alzheimer's.

What to do: If you are thinking about initiating hormone replacement therapy five years or more after the onset of menopause, talk to your doctor about the possible benefits and risks.

4. A Concussion

A study published in *Neurology* in 2012 showed that NFL football players had nearly four times higher risk for Alzheimer's than the general population—no doubt from repeated brain injuries incurred while playing football.

What most people don't realize: Your risk of developing Alzheimer's is doubled if you've ever had a serious concussion that resulted in loss of consciousness—this newer evidence shows that it is crucially important to prevent head injuries of any kind throughout your life.

What to do: Fall-proof your home, with commonsense measures such as adequate lighting, eliminating or securing throw rugs and keeping stairways clear. Wear shoes with firm soles and low heels, which also helps prevent falls.

If you've ever had a concussion, it's important to implement the full range of Alzheimer's-prevention strategies in this article.

5. Not Having a Purpose in Life

In a seven-year study published in *Archives of General Psychiatry*, researchers at the Rush Alzheimer's Disease Center in Chicago found that people who had a "purpose in life" were 2.4 times less likely to develop Alzheimer's.

What to do: The researchers found that the people who agreed with the following statements were less likely to develop Alzheimer's and mild cognitive impairment—"I feel good when I think of what I have done in the past and what I hope to do in the future" and "I have a sense of direction and purpose in life."

If you cannot genuinely agree with the above statements, there are things you can do to change that—in fact, you even can change the way you feel about your past. It takes a bit of resolve…some action…and perhaps help from a qualified mental health counselor.

One way to start: Think about and make a list of some activities that would make your life more meaningful. Ask yourself, Am I doing these?… and then write down small, realistic goals that will involve you more in those activities, such as volunteering one hour every week at a local hospital or signing up for a class at your community college next semester.

The following steps are crucial in the fight against Alzheimer's disease…

- Lose weight if you're overweight.
- Control high blood pressure.
- Exercise regularly.
- Engage in activities that challenge your mind.
- Eat a diet rich in colorful fruits and vegetables and low in saturated fat, such as the Mediterranean diet.
- Take a daily supplement containing 2,000 milligrams of omega-3 fatty acids.

How Not to Worry About Your Memory

Aaron P. Nelson, PhD, chief of neuropsychology in the division of cognitive and behavioral neurology at Brigham and Women's Hospital. He is coauthor, with Susan Gilbert, of *The Harvard Medical School Guide to Achieving Optimal Memory*.

With all the media coverage of Alzheimer's disease and other forms of dementia, it's easy to imagine the worst every time you can't summon the name of a good friend or struggle to remember the details of a novel that you put down just a few days ago.

Reassuring: The minor memory hiccups that bedevil adults in middle age and beyond usually are due to normal changes in the brain and nervous system that affect concentration or the processing and storing of information. In fact, common memory "problems" typically are nothing more than memory errors. Forgetting is just one kind of error.

Important: Memory problems that are frequent or severe (such as forgetting how to drive home from work or how to operate a simple appliance in your home) could be a sign of Alzheimer's disease or some other form of dementia. Such memory lapses also can be due to treatable, but potentially serious, conditions, including depression, a nutritional deficiency or even sleep apnea. See your doctor if you have memory problems that interfere with daily life—or the frequency and/or severity seems to be increasing. Five types of harmless memory errors that tend to get more common with age…

MEMORY ERROR #1: **Absentmindedness.** How many times have you had to search for the car keys because you put them in an entirely unexpected place? Or gone to the grocery store to buy three items but come home with only two? This type of forgetfulness describes what happens when a new piece of information (where you put the keys or what to buy at the store) never even enters your memory because you weren't paying attention.

My advice: Since distraction is the main cause of absentmindedness, try to do just one thing at a time.

Otherwise, here's what can happen: You start to do something, and then something else grabs your attention—and you completely forget about the first thing.

We live in a world in which information routinely comes at us from all directions, so you'll want to develop your own systems for getting things done. There's no good reason to use brain space for superfluous or transitory information. Use lists, sticky notes, e-mail reminders, etc., for tasks, names of books you want to read, grocery lists, etc. There's truth to the Chinese proverb that says, "The palest ink is better than the best memory."

Helpful: Don't write a to-do list and put it aside. While just the act of writing down tasks can help you remember them, you should consult your list several times a day for it to be effective.

MEMORY ERROR #2: **Blocking.** When a word or the answer to a question is "on the tip of your tongue," you're blocking the information that you need. A similar situation happens when you accidentally call one of your children by the name of another. Some patients are convinced that temporarily "forgetting" an acquaintance's name means that they're developing Alzheimer's disease, but that's usually not true.

Blocking occurs when the information that you need is properly stored in memory, but another piece of information is getting in the way. Often, this second piece of information has similar qualities (names of children, closely related words, etc.) to the first. The similarity may cause the wrong brain area to activate and make it harder to access the information that you want.

My advice: Don't get frustrated when a word or name is on the tip of your tongue. Relax and think about something else. In about 50% of cases, the right answer will come to you within one minute.

MEMORY ERROR #3: **Misattribution.** This is what happens when you make a mistake in the source of a memory.

More than a few writers have been embarrassed when they wrote something that they thought was original but later learned that it was identical to something they had heard or read. You might tell a story to friends that you know is true because you read about it in the newspaper—except that you may have only heard people talking about it and misattributed the source.

Misattribution happens more frequently with age because older people have older memories. These memories are more likely to contain mistakes because they happened long ago and don't get recalled often.

My advice: Concentrate on details when you want to remember the source of information.

Focus on the five Ws: Who told you…what the content was…when it happened…where you were when you learned it…and why it's important. Asking these questions will help to strengthen the context of the information.

MEMORY ERROR #4: Suggestibility. Most individuals think of memory as a mental videotape—a recording of what took place. But what feels like memories to you could be things that never really happened. Memories can be affected or even created by the power of suggestion.

In a landmark study, researchers privately asked the relatives of participants to describe three childhood events that actually happened. They were also asked to provide plausible details about a fourth scenario (getting lost in a shopping mall) that could have happened but didn't.

A few weeks later, the participants were given a written description of the four stories and asked to recall them in as much detail as possible. They weren't told that one of the stories was fictional.

What happened: About 20% of the participants believed that they really had been lost in a shopping mall. They "remembered" the event and provided details about what happened. This and other studies show that memories can be influenced—and even created—from thin air.

My advice: Keep an open mind if your memory of an event isn't the same as someone else's. It's unlikely that either of you will have perfect recall. Memories get modified over time by new information as well as by individual perspectives, personality traits, etc.

MEMORY ERROR #5: Transience. You watched a great movie but can't remember the lead actor two hours later. You earned an advanced degree in engineering, but now you can hardly remember the basic equations.

These are all examples of transience, the tendency of memories to fade over time. Short-term memory is highly susceptible to transience because information that you've just acquired hasn't been embedded in long-term storage, where memories can be more stable and enduring.

This is why you're more likely to forget the name of someone you just met than the details of a meaningful book that you read in college—although even long-term memories will fade if you do not recall them now and then.

My advice: You need to rehearse and revisit information in order to retain it. Repeating a name several times after you've met someone is a form of rehearsal. So is talking about a movie you just watched or jotting notes about an event in a diary.

Revisiting information simply means recalling and using it. Suppose that you wrote down your thoughts about an important conversation in your journal. You can review the notes a few weeks later to strengthen the memory and anchor it in your mind. The same technique will help you remember names, telephone numbers, etc.

Memory Robbers That Are Often Overlooked

Cynthia Green, PhD, a clinical psychologist, author and one of America's foremost experts on brain health. She is founding director of The Memory Enhancement Program at Icahn School of Medicine at Mount Sinai, New York City, and president and CEO of Total Brain Health and TBH Brands, LLC, in Montclair, New Jersey. CynthiaGreenPhD.com

Alzheimer's disease is such a dreaded diagnosis that you may be filled with panic if you experience occasional memory loss. But these worries may be unnecessary.

As people age, the brain undergoes changes that may lead to some decline in short-term memory. This is normal.

Of course memory loss that truly concerns you is another matter. Ask your primary care physician to refer you to a neurologist or geriatrician for an evaluation if...

•**You have noticed a significant change in your everyday memory over the past six months.**

•**Friends or family members have expressed concern about your memory.**

•**You have begun forgetting recent conversations.**

In the meantime, consider whether your occasional forgetfulness may be due to one of the following causes, all of which can be easily corrected...

Not Enough Sleep

Poor sleep is probably the most common cause of occasional memory lapses. The ability to concentrate suffers with insufficient rest. Sleep also appears to be essential for consolidating memory—whatever information you learn during the day, whether it's the name of a colleague or the street where a new restaurant opened, you need sleep to make it stick in your mind.

Self-defense: If you're not sleeping seven to eight hours nightly, make it a priority to get more sleep. If you are unable to improve your sleep on your own, talk to your doctor.

Widely Used Drugs

Impaired memory is a potential side effect of many medications. Obvious suspects include prescription sleeping pills...opiate painkillers, such as *meperidine* (Demerol)...and anti-anxiety drugs, such as *diazepam* (Valium) and *alprazolam* (Xanax).

Certain blood pressure–lowering medications, such as beta-blockers, and antidepressants also cause memory problems in some people. Even over-the-counter antihistamines, such as *diphenhydramine* (Benadryl), can have this effect.

If you're taking multiple medications, more than one may cause impaired memory, making it even more difficult to identify the culprit.

Timing is often a tip-off: When impaired memory is an adverse drug effect, it's most likely to appear when you start taking a new medication or increase the dose. But not always.

As we grow older, our bodies become less efficient at clearing medications from the body, so the same dose you've been taking safely for years may cause problems you never had before.

Self-defense: If you think medication might be affecting your memory, do not stop taking the drug or reduce the dosage on your own. Talk to your doctor or pharmacist for advice.

Emotional Upset

When you're anxious, stressed or depressed, your ability to concentrate suffers. Whatever it is that worries or preoccupies you keeps your mind from focusing on facts, names, faces and places, so they aren't absorbed into memory.

Self-defense: To keep everyday tensions from undercutting your memory, practice some form of relaxation or stress reduction. Yoga, meditation, deep breathing—or something as simple as allowing yourself a soothing time-out to walk or chat with a friend—can relieve accumulated stress and bolster your recall.

True depression is something else: Even mild-to-moderate depression can sap your energy, take pleasure out of life and affect your memory. If you suspect that you may be depressed, be alert for other symptoms—such as difficulty sleeping, sadness, apathy and a negative outlook—and see your doctor or a mental-health professional.

Too Much Alcohol

Moderate red wine consumption has been shown to promote the health of your heart and arteries. Because of this cardiovascular health benefit, red wine also may reduce risk for dementia.

Excessive drinking, on the other hand, is harmful to the brain. Among its devastating toxic effects is a severe and often irreversible form of memory loss called Korsakoff's syndrome, a condition that occurs in alcoholics.

Alcohol's effect on memory can be subtle. Some people find that even a glass or two of wine daily is enough to interfere with learning facts and recalling information. Pay attention to how mentally sharp you feel after having a drink. If you think your alcohol intake may be causing forgetfulness, cut back. Remember, tolerance for alcohol generally declines with age, giving the same drink more impact.

Self-defense: There is more scientific evidence supporting red wine's brain-protective effect than for any other form of alcohol. If you are a man, do not exceed two glasses of red wine daily, and if you are a woman, limit yourself to one glass daily.

Illness

A simple cold or headache is enough to interfere with your concentration and recall.

Illnesses that commonly go undiagnosed also may play a role. For example, when the thyroid gland (which regulates metabolism) is underactive, the mind slows down along with the body. (Other signs of an underactive thyroid include weight gain, constipation, thin or brittle hair and depression.) An overactive thyroid can affect your memory by making you anxious, "wired" and easily distracted.

Memory impairment also may be a symptom of other disorders, such as Parkinson's disease, multiple sclerosis or Lyme disease.

Nutritional Deficiency

An easily overlooked memory robber is a vitamin B-12 deficiency, often marked by general fatigue and slowed thinking. Older people are especially at risk—as we age, our ability to absorb vitamin B-12 from foods diminishes.

Self-defense: If you have occasional memory lapses, ask your doctor for a blood test to check your vitamin B-12 level.

Safeguarding Your Memory: Control Chronic Health Issues

Studies have shown repeatedly that people with high blood pressure, athero-sclerosis (fatty buildup in the arteries), obesity and/or diabetes are at dramatically increased risk of developing dementia in their later years.

The effect of these chronic medical conditions on day-to-day memory is less clear. Research shows that memory declines when blood sugar rises in people with diabetes and improves when they take dietary steps to stabilize it.

Self-defense: If you have a chronic health problem, work with your doctor to keep your symptoms under control.

Best Workouts to Keep Your Brain "Buff"

Cynthia Green, PhD, a clinical psychologist, author and one of America's foremost experts on brain health. She is founding director of The Memory Enhancement Program at Icahn School of Medicine at Mount Sinai, New York City, and president and CEO of Total Brain Health and TBH Brands, LLC, in Montclair, New Jersey. CynthiaGreen PhD.com

We all want to keep our brains in top shape. But are crossword puzzles, online classes and the other such activities that we've been hearing about for years the best ways to do that? Not really.

Now: To improve memory and preserve overall cognitive function, the latest research reveals that it takes more than quiet puzzle-solving and streaming lectures.

Even more intriguing: Some activities that we once thought were time wasters may actually help build intellectual capacity and other cognitive functions.

Here are effective ways to keep your brain "buff"...

A Healthy Brain

The most important steps to keep your brain performing at optimal levels are lifestyle choices...

- **Getting aerobic exercise (at least 150 minutes per week).**
- **Maintaining a healthy body weight.**
- **Not smoking.**
- **Eating a diet that emphasizes fruits and vegetables and is low in refined sugar and white flour**—two of the biggest dietary threats to brain health that have recently been identified by researchers.

Additional benefits are possible with regular brain workouts. In the past, experts thought that nearly any game or activity that challenges you to think would improve your general brain functioning.

What research now tells us: An increasing body of evidence shows that improved memory requires something more—you need to work against a clock. Games with a time limit force you to think quickly and with agility. These are the factors that lead to improved memory and mental focus. Among my favorite brain workouts—aim for at least 30 minutes daily of any combination of the activities below...

Brainy Computer Games

Specialized brain-training computer programs (such as Lumosity, Fit Brains and CogniFit) are no longer the darlings of the health community. Formerly marketed as a fun way to reduce one's risk for dementia, recent evidence has not supported that claim.

These programs do provide, however, a variety of activities that may help improve intellectual performance, attention, memory and mental flexibility. Lumosity and other programs are a good option for people who enjoy a regimented brain workout, including such activities as remembering sequences and ignoring distractions. Monthly prices range from $4.99 to $19.95.

Other options to consider trying...

•**Action video games.** These games were once considered "brain-numbing" activities that kept players from developing intellectual and social skills. Recent research, however, shows that action video games can promote mental focus, flexible thinking, and decision-making and problem-solving skills. Because these games are timed, they also require quick responses from the players.

Good choices: World of Warcraft, The Elder Scrolls and Guild Wars, all of which involve role-playing by assuming the identity of various characters to battle foes and complete quests, often with other virtual players. These games are available in DVD format for Mac or PC and with an online subscription for virtual play.

Caveat: An hour or two can be a brain booster, but don't overdo it. Too much role-playing takes you away from real-life interactions.

•**Free brain-boosting computer game for a cause.** At FreeRice.com, you can answer fun and challenging questions in such subjects as English vocabulary, foreign languages, math and humanities. With each correct answer, the United Nations World Food Programme donates 10 grains of rice to a Third World country. To date, players have "earned" a total of nearly 100 billion grains of rice—enough to create more than 10 million meals.

To increase the challenge: Set a timer so that you must work against the clock.

Apps for Your Brain

If you'd prefer to use an "app"—a software application that you can use on a smartphone or similar electronic device—there are several good options. *Among the best fun/challenging apps (free on Android and Apple)…*

•**Words with Friends.** This ever-popular game allows you to play a Scrabble-like game against your friends who have also downloaded the app on an electronic device. The game provides even more benefits if it's used with the time-clock feature.

•**Word Streak with Friends** (formerly Scramble with Friends) is a timed find-a-word game. You can play on your own or with friends.

•**Elevate** was named Apple's Best App of 2014. It provides a structured game environment that feels more like a test, focusing on reading, writing and math skills, than a game. Still, this timed app will give Apple users a good brain challenge.

Tech-free Options

If you'd rather not stare at the screen of a computer or some other electronic device for your brain workout, here are some good options…

• **Tech-free games.** SET is a fast-paced card game that tests your visual perception skills. Players race to find a set of three matching cards (based on color, shape, number or shading) from an array of cards placed on a table.

Bonus: This game can be played by one player or as many people as can fit around the table. The winner of dozens of "Best Game" awards, including the high-IQ group Mensa's Select award, SET is fun for kids and adults alike.

Another good choice: Boggle, which challenges you to create words from a given set of letter cubes within a three-minute period. It can be played by two or more people.

• **Drumming.** Playing any musical instrument requires attention and a keen sense of timing. Basic drumming is a great activity for beginner musicians (especially if you don't have the finger dexterity for piano or guitar).

Even better: Join a drumming circle, which provides the extra challenge of matching your timing and rhythm to the rest of the drummers, along with opportunities for socialization.

Bonus: Research has demonstrated that some forms, such as African djembe drumming, count as a low- to moderate-intensity activity that may reduce blood pressure, which helps protect the brain from blood vessel damage.

• **Meditation.** This practice improves cognitive function and sensory processing and promotes mental focus. Meditating for about 30 minutes daily has also been linked to greater blood flow to the brain and increased gray matter (associated with positive emotions, memory and decision-making). The benefits have even been seen among some people with early-stage neurodegenerative diseases, such as Alzheimer's disease.

A good way to get started: Begin with a simple "mindful eating" exercise— spend the first five minutes of each meal really focusing on what you're eating. Don't talk, read the paper or watch TV…just savor the food. Eventually, you'll want to expand this level of attention to other parts of your day. Such mindfulness habits are a good complement to a regular meditation practice.

• **Coloring.** If you have kids or grandkids, don't just send them off with their crayons. Color with them.

Even better: Get one of the new breed of coloring books with complex designs for adults. While there hasn't been specific research addressing the brain benefits of coloring, this form of play has been shown to reduce stress in children, and it is thought to boost creativity and have a meditative quality. You can find coloring books made for adults at bookstores and art-supply stores.

The Diet That Cuts Your Alzheimer's Risk in Half

Martha Clare Morris, ScD, professor and director of the Section of Nutrition and Nutritional Epidemiology at Rush University, Chicago, where she is assistant provost for community research. She specializes in dietary and other preventable risk factors in the development of Alzheimer's disease and other chronic diseases in older adults.

The MIND diet blends components from DASH (a blood pressure–lowering diet) and the popular Mediterranean diet, with an extra emphasis on berries, leafy greens and a few other brain-healthy foods.

How good is it? People who carefully followed the diet were about 53% less likely to develop Alzheimer's disease in subsequent years. Those who approached it more casually didn't do quite as well but still reduced their risk considerably, by about 35%.

Blended Benefits

The MIND diet was developed by researchers at Rush University who examined years of studies to identify specific foods and nutrients that seemed to be particularly good—or bad—for long-term brain health. The MIND (it stands for Mediterranean-DASH Intervention for Neurodegenerative Delay) diet is a hybrid plan that incorporates the "best of the best."

In a study in the journal *Alzheimer's & Dementia*, the researchers followed more than 900 participants. None had dementia when the study started. The participants filled out food questionnaires and had repeated neurological tests over a period averaging more than four years.

Some participants followed the MIND diet. Others followed the older DASH diet or the Mediterranean diet. All three diets reduced the risk for Alzheimer's disease. But only the MIND diet did so even when the participants followed the plan only "moderately well."

The MIND diet specifies "brain-healthy" food groups and five groups that need to be limited, either eaten in moderation or preferably not at all.

What to Eat

•**More leafy greens.** Kale really is a superfood for the brain. So are spinach, chard, beet greens and other dark, leafy greens. The Mediterranean and DASH diets advise people to eat more vegetables, but they don't specify which ones.

The MIND diet specifically recommends one serving of greens a day, in addition to one other vegetable. Previous research has shown that a vegetable-rich diet can help prevent cognitive decline, but two of the larger studies found that leafy greens were singularly protective.

•**Lots of nuts.** The diet calls for eating nuts five times a week. Nuts are high in vitamin E and monounsaturated and polyunsaturated fats—all good for brain health.

The study didn't look at which nuts were more likely to be beneficial. Eating a variety is probably a good idea because you'll get a varied mix of protective nutrients and antioxidants. Raw or roasted nuts are fine (as long as they're not roasted in fat and highly salted). If you are allergic to nuts, seeds such as sunflower and pumpkin seeds are good sources of these nutrients as well.

•**Berries.** These are the only fruits that are specifically included in the MIND diet. Other fruits are undoubtedly good for you, but none has been shown in studies to promote cognitive health. Berries, on the other hand, have been shown to slow age-related cognitive decline. In laboratory studies, a berry-rich diet improves memory and protects against abnormal changes in the brain. Blueberries seem to be particularly potent. Eat berries at least twice a week.

•**Beans and whole grains.** These fiber-rich and folate-rich foods provide high levels of protein with much less saturated fat than you would get from an equivalent helping of meat. The MIND diet calls for three daily servings of whole grains and three weekly servings of beans.

•**Include fish and poultry—but you don't need to go overboard.** Seafood is a key component of the Mediterranean diet, and some proponents recommend eating it four times a week or more. The MIND diet calls for only one weekly serving, although more is OK. A once-a-week fish meal is enough for brain health.

There is no data to specify the number of poultry servings needed for brain health, but we recommend two servings a week.

•**A glass of wine.** People who drink no wine—or those who drink too much—are more likely to suffer cognitive declines than those who drink just a little.

Recommended: One glass a day. Red wine, in particular, is high in flavonoids and polyphenols that may be protective for the brain.

Foods to Limit

•**Limit red meat, cheese, butter and margarine**—along with fast food, fried food and pastries and other sweets. The usual suspects, in other words.

All of these food groups increase the risk for Alzheimer's disease, probably because of their high levels of saturated fat (or, in the case of some margarines, trans fats). Saturated fat has been linked to higher cholesterol, more systemic inflammation and possibly a disruption of the blood-brain barrier that may allow harmful substances into the brain.

However, most nutritionists acknowlege the importance of letting people enjoy some treats and not being so restrictive that they give up eating healthfully altogether.

Try to follow these recommendations…

Red meat: No more than three servings a week.

Butter and margarine: Less than one tablespoon daily. Cook with olive oil instead.

Cheese: Less than one serving a week.

Pastries and sweets: Yes, you can enjoy some treats, but limit yourself to five servings or fewer a week.

Fried or fast food: Less than one serving a week.

Supplements That Stop Memory Loss

Pamela Wartian Smith, MD, MPH, codirector of the master's program in medical sciences with a concentration in metabolic and nutritional medicine at Morsani College of Medicine at University of South Florida. She is author of *What You Must Know About Memory Loss & How You Can Stop It: A Guide to Proven Techniques and Supplements to Maintain, Strengthen, or Regain Memory.* CenterforPersonalizedMedicine.com

Mild forgetfulness, known as age-related memory impairment, is a natural part of getting older. By age 75, a person's memory has declined, on average, by about 43%. After age 75, the hippocampus, the part of the brain most closely associated with memory, will eventually atrophy at the rate of 1% to 2% each year.

But you can improve memory with over-the-counter supplements—if you choose the right ones. Here are the supplements I find most effective with my patients. You can take several of these if you choose. You could start with phosphatidylserine and add others depending on your personal needs. For example, if you're taking a medication that depletes CoQ10, you might want to take that supplement. Or if you're under stress, add ashwagandha root. Of course, always check with your doctor before starting any new supplement.

•**Phosphatidylserine (PS).** Most people haven't heard of it, but PS is one of my first choices for mild memory loss. It's a naturally occurring phospholipid (a molecule that contains two fatty acids) that increases the body's production of acetylcholine and other neurotransmitters. It improves cell-to-cell communication and "nourishes" the brain by improving glucose metabolism.

Studies have shown that healthy people who take PS are more likely to maintain their ability to remember things. For those who have already experienced age-related memory loss, PS can improve memory. It's also thought to improve symptoms caused by some forms of dementia.

Typical dose: 300 mg daily. You're unlikely to notice any side effects.

•**Co-enzyme Q10 (CoQ10).** This is another naturally occurring substance found in many foods (such as fatty fish, meats, nuts, fruits and vegetables) and in nearly all of your body's tissues. CoQ10 increases the production of adenosine triphosphate, a molecule that enhances energy production within cells. It's also a potent antioxidant that reduces cell-damaging inflammation in the brain and other parts of the body.

People with degenerative brain disorders, such as Alzheimer's, tend to have lower levels of CoQ10. Studies suggest that supplemental CoQ10 improves memory by protecting brain cells from oxidative damage.

Important: If you're taking a medication that depletes CoQ10—examples include statins (for lowering cholesterol)…metformin (for diabetes)…and beta-blockers (for heart disease and other conditions)—you'll definitely want to take a supplement. I often recommend it for people age 50 and older because the body's production of CoQ10 declines with age. Hard exercise also depletes it.

Typical dose: Between 30 mg and 360 mg daily. Ask your health-care professional how much you need—it will depend on medication use and other factors. Side effects are rare but may include insomnia, agitation and digestive problems such as diarrhea and heartburn.

●**Acetyl-L-carnitine.** A study that looked at people with mild cognitive impairment (an intermediate stage between age-related memory impairment and dementia) found that acetyl-L-carnitine improved memory, attention and even verbal fluency.

Acetyl-L-carnitine (it is derived from an amino acid) is a versatile molecule. It's used by the body to produce acetylcholine, the main neurotransmitter involved in memory. It slows the rate of neurotransmitter decay, increases oxygen availability and helps convert body fat into energy.

Typical dose: 1,000 mg to 2,000 mg daily. Check with your health-care professional before starting acetyl-L-carnitine to see what dose is best for you. If your kidneys are not functioning perfectly, you may need a lower dose. Some people may notice a slight fishy body odor. In my experience, you can prevent this by taking 50 mg to 100 mg of vitamin B-2 at the same time you take acetyl-L-carnitine.

●**Ashwagandha root.** This is an herb that improves the repair and regeneration of brain cells (neurons) and inhibits the body's production of acetylcholinesterase, an enzyme that degrades acetylcholine. It also improves the ability to deal with both physical and emotional stress—both of which have been linked to impaired memory and cognitive decline.

Typical dose: 500 mg to 2,000 mg daily. Start with the lower dose. If after a month you don't notice that your memory and focus have improved, take a little more. GI disturbances are possible but not common.

Warning: Don't take this supplement if you're also taking a prescription medication that has cholinesterase-inhibiting effects, such as *donepezil* (Aricept) or *galantamine* (Razadyne). Ask your health-care professional whether any of your medications have this effect.

●**Ginkgo biloba.** Among the most studied herbal supplements, ginkgo is an antioxidant that protects the hippocampus from age-related atrophy. It's a vasodilator that helps prevent blood clots, improves brain circulation and reduces the risk for vascular dementia, a type of dementia associated with impaired blood flow to the brain. It also increases the effects of serotonin, a neurotransmitter that's involved in mood and learning.

Bonus: In animal studies, ginkgo appears to block the formation of amyloid, the protein that has been linked to Alzheimer's disease. There's strong evidence that ginkgo can stabilize and possibly improve memory.

Typical dose: 60 mg to 120 mg daily. Most people won't have side effects, but ginkgo is a blood thinner that can react with other anticoagulants. If you're taking *warfarin* or another blood thinner (including aspirin and fish oil), be sure to check with your health-care professional before taking ginkgo.

•**Fish oil.** Much of the brain consists of DHA (docosahexaenoic acid), one of the main omega-3 fatty acids. It is essential for brain health. People who take fish-oil supplements have improved brain circulation and a faster transmission of nerve signals.

Studies have found that people who eat a lot of fatty fish have a lower risk for mild cognitive impairment than people who tend to eat little or no fatty fish. One study found that people with age-related memory impairment achieved better scores on memory tests when they took daily DHA supplements.

Typical dose: 2,000 mg daily if you're age 50 or older. Look for a combination supplement that includes equal amounts of DHA and EPA (another omega-3). Fish-oil supplements can increase the effects of blood-thinning medications such as aspirin and warfarin if the dose is above 3,000 mg a day.

•**Huperzine A.** Extracted from a Chinese moss, this is a cholinesterase inhibitor that increases brain levels of acetylcholine. It also protects brain cells from too-high levels of glutamate, another neurotransmitter.

Huperzine A may improve memory and could even help delay symptoms of Alzheimer's disease. A study conducted by the National Institute of Aging found that patients with mild-to-moderate Alzheimer's who took huperzine A had improvements in cognitive functions.

Recommended dose: 400 mcg daily. Don't take it if you're already taking a prescription cholinesterase inhibitor (as discussed in the "Ashwagandha root" section).

CHAPTER 12

Heart Health and Stroke

14 Little Things You Can Do for a Healthier Heart

Joel K. Kahn, MD, clinical professor of medicine at Wayne State University School of Medicine, Detroit, and founder of The Kahn Center for Cardiac Longevity. He is author of *The Whole Heart Solution: Halt Heart Disease Now with the Best Alternative and Traditional Medicine.* DrJoelKahn.com

Heart disease is America's number-one killer. But just because it's a major health risk does not necessarily mean that you must make major lifestyle changes to avoid it. *Here are 14 simple and inexpensive ways to have a healthier heart...*

Doable Diet Tips

1. Don't eat in the evening. Research suggests that the heart (and digestive system) benefits greatly from taking an 11-to-12-hour break from food every night. One study found that men who indulge in midnight snacks are 55% more likely to suffer from heart disease than men who don't. So if you plan to eat breakfast at 7 am, consider your kitchen closed after 7 or 8 pm.

Warning: You cannot produce the same health benefits by snacking at night and then skipping breakfast. This might create an 11-to-12-hour break from eating, but skipping breakfast actually increases the risk for heart attack and/or death—by 27%, according to one study. Our bodies and minds often are under considerable stress in the morning—that's when heart attack risk is greatest. Skipping the morning meal only adds to this stress.

2. Use apple pie spice as a topping on oatmeal and fruit. Some people enjoy it in coffee, too. This spice combo, which contains cinnamon, cloves, nutmeg and allspice, has been shown to reduce blood pressure, improve cholesterol levels and lower the risk for heart disease.

3. Take your time with your tea. Tea contains compounds called flavonoids that have been shown to significantly reduce the risk for heart disease—green tea is best of all. But you get the full benefits only if you have the patience to let the tea leaves steep—that is, soak in hot water—for at least three to five minutes before drinking.

4. Fill up on salad. It's no secret that being overweight is bad for the heart. But most people don't realize that they can lose weight without going hungry. Salad can make the stomach feel full without a lot of calories. But don't add nonvegetable ingredients such as cheese, meat and egg to salads…and opt for balsamic or red wine vinegar dressing—they are rich in nutrients, including artery-healing resveratrol.

As a bonus, vegetables…and fruits…contain nutrients that are great for the heart regardless of your weight—so great that eating a plant-rich diet could improve your blood pressure just as much as taking blood pressure medication. In fact, one study found that increasing consumption of fruits and vegetables from 1.5 to eight servings per day decreases the risk for heart attack or stroke by 30%.

One strategy: Become a vegetarian for breakfast and lunch. That way you still can enjoy meat at dinner, but your overall vegetable consumption will be increased.

5. Marinate meat before grilling it. Grilling meat triggers a dramatic increase in its "advanced glycation end products" (AGEs), which stiffen blood vessels and raise blood pressure, among other health drawbacks. If you're not willing to give up your grill, marinate meat for at least 30 minutes before cooking it. Marinating helps keep meat moist, which can slash AGE levels in half. An effective marinade for this purpose is beer, though lemon juice or vinegar works well, too. You can add herbs and oil if you wish.

6. Sprinkle Italian seasoning mix onto salads, potatoes and soups. This zesty mix contains antioxidant-rich herbs such as oregano, sage, rosemary and thyme, which studies suggest reduce the risk for heart disease and cancer.

7. Avoid foods that contain dangerous additives. There are so many food additives that it's virtually impossible to keep track of them all. Focus on avoiding foods that list any of the following seven among their ingredients—each carries heart-related health risks. The seven are aspartame…BHA (butylated hydroxyanisole)…BHT (butylated hydroxytoluene)…saccharin…sodium nitrate…sodium sulfate…and monosodium glutamate (MSG).

8. Savor the first three bites of everything you eat. When people eat too fast, they also tend to eat too much. One way to slow down your eating is to force yourself to pay close attention to what you are eating. If you cannot do this for an entire meal or snack, at least do it for the first three mouthfuls of each food you consume. Chew these initial bites slowly and thoroughly. Give the food and its flavor your undivided attention, and you will end up eating less.

9. Prepare your lunch the night before if you won't be home for your midday meal. People who intend to make their lunch in the morning often are in too much of a rush to do so…then wind up resorting to fast food.

10. Buy organic when it counts. Higher pesticide levels in the blood predict higher cholesterol levels as well as cardiovascular disease. Organic food is free of pesticide—but it can be expensive. The smart compromise is to buy organic when it counts most—when traditionally grown produce is most likely to contain pesticide residue. According to the Environmental Working Group, the foods most likely to contain pesticide residue are apples, celery, cherry tomatoes, collard greens, cucumbers, grapes, hot peppers, kale, nectarines, peaches, potatoes, spinach, strawberries, summer squash and sweet bell peppers.

Important: If your options are eating conventionally farmed fruits and vegetables or not eating fruits and vegetables at all, definitely consume the conventionally grown produce. The health risks from small amounts of pesticide residue are much lower than the health risks from not eating produce.

Easy Lifestyle Habits

11. Stand two to five minutes each hour. Recent research suggests that sitting for extended periods is horrible for your heart. Sitting slows your metabolism and reduces your ability to process glucose and cholesterol. But standing for as little as two to five minutes each hour seems to significantly reduce these health consequences (more standing is even better). Stand while making phone calls or during commercials. Buy a "standing desk," then stand when you use your computer.

12. Take walks after meals. Walking is good anytime, but walks after meals have special health benefits, particularly after rich desserts. A 20-minute postmeal stroll significantly improves the body's ability to manage blood sugar. Maintaining healthful blood sugar levels reduces risk for coronary artery blockage.

13. Exercise in brief but intense bursts. Research suggests that exercising as intensely as possible for 20 seconds…resting for 10 seconds…then repeating this seven more times provides nearly the same benefits for the heart as a far longer but less intense workout. Try this with an exercise bike, rowing machine, elliptical machine or any other form of exercise. Do an Internet search for "Tabata training" to learn more. There are free apps that can help you time these intervals. Download Tabata Stopwatch in the iTunes store if you use an Apple device…or Tabata Timer for HIIT from Google Play if you use an Android device.

Caution: Talk to your doctor. High-intensity training could be dangerous if you have a preexisting health condition.

14. Get sufficient sleep. One study found that the rates of heart disease for people who get seven to eight hours of sleep a night are nearly half those of people who get too little or too much sleep.

Heart-Rhythm Problem? These Supplements Can Help

Michael Traub, ND, director, Ho'o Lokahi, an integrative health care center in Kailua Kona, Hawaii.

The occasional flutter…a missed beat…an unusual thump. For some people, an irregularity in heartbeat, called cardiac arrhythmia, signals only a minor glitch in the heart's complex internal electrical system. But in other cases, it indicates a serious electrical malfunction that can lead to atrial fibrillation, an abnormally fast and irregular heartbeat—and that can in turn be associated with heart failure, stroke or even sudden death.

Good news: In many cases, nutritional deficiencies cause or contribute to arrhythmias—and addressing those deficiencies with the appropriate dietary supplements can help correct or minimize the heart problem!

To find out whether nutritional therapies are right for you, consult a naturopathic physician or a functional medical doctor experienced in treating arrhythmias. One of the doctor's first steps may be to order blood tests to see what's going on inside your body at the micronutrient level—because your levels of certain nutrients can have a direct impact on your heart rhythm.

For patients with cardiac arrhythmias, it's especially important to check for deficiencies of magnesium and potassium…and the ratio between the omega-6 fatty acid arachidonic acid and the omega-3 fatty acid eicosapentaenoic acid (EPA), because too high a ratio is bad for your heart. You should also be tested for the amino acid homocysteine because high levels are associated with increased risk for heart disease and arrhythmias.

The two most common deficiencies in patients with arrhythmias are magnesium and EPA. Potassium deficiency is not as common, but your potassium level should be checked because deficiency is associated with higher risk for atrial fibrillation.

Rhythm-Regulating Supplements

Based on your blood test results, your doctor will prescribe the appropriate supplements in the proper dosages to correct your nutritional deficiencies and address other factors that can contribute to arrhythmias. *The supplements I typically prescribe for my arrhythmia patients include one or more of the following…*

•**Magnesium.** This mineral relaxes blood vessel walls and improves blood flow. Magnesium is so effective at helping regulate heart rhythm that it is often given to patients in the hospital to reduce the risk for atrial fibrillation and cardiac arrest.

•**Potassium.** This is known to improve and stabilize the pumping action of the heart. It protects against ventricular and atrial fibrillation…it also is used as a treatment for congestive heart failure.

•**Fish oil.** Several years ago, some studies showed that omega-3 fatty acids reduced fatal ventricular arrhythmias, although more recent studies have not confirmed these findings. Still, because omega-3 fatty acids have a positive effect on heart health, fish oil is an important part of a natural anti-arrhythmia regimen.

Caution: Since fish oil is an anticoagulant, its use must be medically supervised in patients who take blood-thinning medication.

●**Lumbrokinase.** This enzyme is similar to the better-known nattokinase (made from fermented soybeans). Lumbrokinase is derived from the earthworm *Lumbricus rubellus*—but don't be put off by that, because it works even better than nattokinase to inhibit the formation of blood clots. Like fish oil, lumbrokinase should be taken only with a doctor's OK by anyone who is on a pharmaceutical blood thinner.

●**Hawthorn.** This herb contains antioxidants that are thought to improve blood flow.

●**B vitamins.** If your homocysteine levels are high, your doctor may prescribe supplements of vitamins B-6, B-12 and/or B-9 (folate) to bring your levels into normal range.

What to avoid: Patients with arrhythmias should not take iodine supplements because they can bring about hyperthyroidism, which worsens arrhythmia. Caffeine—whether from food, beverages or supplements—also should be avoided because the stimulant can interfere with heart rhythms.

Also helpful for arrhythmia patients: It's best to limit alcohol intake...not smoke...get enough sleep...stay adequately hydrated...eat plenty of fresh fruits and vegetables...and take steps to effectively manage stress. These lifestyle choices can make a significant difference when it comes to easing arrhythmias.

Foods That Help Control Blood Pressure

Janet Bond Brill, PhD, RD, a registered dietitian and a nationally recognized expert in nutrition and cardiovascular disease prevention. She is the author of *Blood Pressure Down: The 10-Step Plan to Lower Your Blood Pressure in 4 Weeks Without Prescription Drugs.* DrJanet.com

Mark Houston, MD, MS, director of the Hypertension Institute, Vascular Biology and the Life Extension Institute at Saint Thomas Hospital in Nashville. He is author of *What Your Doctor May Not Tell You About Hypertension.*

Considering all the dangers of high blood pressure (including increased risk for heart attack, stroke and dementia), we definitely want to do everything we can to keep our blood pressure levels under control. But are we?

Unfortunately, one surprisingly simple step—eating the right foods—consistently gets ignored as an effective technique for controlling blood pressure.*

*In addition to smart eating habits, a blood pressure–controlling action plan includes regular exercise (ideally, 30 minutes of aerobic activity, such as brisk walking or swimming, at least five times a week) and a stress-reducing regimen.

Of course everyone knows that a low-sodium diet helps some people maintain healthy blood pressure levels. But there's a lot more to blood pressure control than avoiding that bag of potato chips, extra dash of soy sauce or a crunchy dill pickle (just one dill pickle contains about 875 mg of sodium, or nearly 40% of recommended daily sodium intake).

What most people are missing out on: With the right combination of blood pressure–controlling nutrients, you often can avoid high blood pressure altogether…or if you already have the condition and are being treated with medication, you may be able to reduce your dosage and curb your risk for troubling side effects, such as fatigue, depression and erectile dysfunction.

The best foods for blood pressure control…

Eat More Bananas

Bananas are among the best sources of potassium, a mineral that's crucial for blood pressure control. A typical banana contains about 450 mg of potassium, or about 10% of the amount of potassium most people should aim for each day.

Potassium works like a "water pill." It's a natural diuretic that enables the kidneys to excrete more sodium while also relaxing blood vessels—both functions help control blood pressure.

Scientific evidence: In a large study of nearly 250,000 adults published in the *Journal of the American College of Cardiology*, people who increased their intake of potassium by 1,600 mg daily were 21% less likely to suffer a stroke than those who ate less.

Kiwifruit also is a concentrated source of potassium with more than 200 mg in each small fruit.

Recommended daily amount of potassium: 4,700 mg. A good potassium-rich breakfast is oatmeal made with soy milk (300 mg), one cup of cantaloupe (430 mg), one cup of fresh-squeezed orange juice (496 mg) and one cup of coffee (116 mg).

Other good potassium sources: Potatoes (purple potatoes have the most), avocados, pistachios and Swiss chard.

Good rule of thumb: To control blood pressure, try to consume three times more potassium than sodium.

Pile On the Spinach

Even if you eat plenty of bananas, all of that potassium won't lower your blood pressure unless you also get enough magnesium. It is estimated that about two-thirds of Americans are deficient in magnesium—and while magnesium supplements might help in some ways, they do not reduce blood pressure. Only magnesium from food—such as spinach, nuts, legumes and oatmeal—offers this benefit due to the nutrient's synergistic effect.

Recommended daily amount of magnesium: 500 mg. One cup of cooked spinach provides 157 mg of magnesium.

Also good: Two ounces of dry-roasted almonds (160 mg).

Dip into Yogurt

Calcium helps the body maintain mineral balance that regulates blood pressure. Calcium also contains a protein that works like a natural ACE inhibitor (one of the most common types of blood pressure medications) and prevents the constriction of blood vessels that raises blood pressure.

Important: Stick to low-fat or no-fat yogurt, milk and cheese—the saturated fat in whole-fat dairy products appears to cancel the blood pressure–lowering effects. In addition, opt for "plain" yogurt to avoid the added sugar that's found in many brands of yogurt. If you don't like the taste of plain yogurt, add a little granola, honey, nuts, seeds, fresh berries or banana.

For a tasty "pumpkin pie" snack: Add plain canned pumpkin, walnuts, pumpkin pie spice and Splenda to plain yogurt and top it with fat-free whipped cream.

Other high-calcium foods: Leafy greens and sardines (with the bones). Calcium supplements also can help keep blood pressure down, but recent research has linked them to increased cardiovascular risk. Talk to your doctor about these supplements.

Recommended daily amount of calcium: 1,000 mg for men age 51 to 70…1,200 mg for men age 71 and older, and women age 51 and older. Eating two fat-free yogurts (830 mg), one cup of cooked spinach (245 mg) and three kiwifruits (150 mg) will easily get you to your daily calcium goal.

Enjoy Soy

Soy foods, including tofu, soy nuts and soy milk, may be the most underrated blood pressure–lowering foods. Research shows that people who regularly eat soy can reduce their blood pressure as much as they would by taking some medications. Soy increases nitric oxide, a naturally occurring gas that lowers blood pressure.

Helpful: If you can't get used to the taste (or texture) of tofu, drink chocolate soy milk. An eight-ounce glass has 8 g of soy protein. Unsalted, dry-roasted soy nuts are an even richer source with about 10 g in a quarter cup.

Recommended daily amount of soy: 20 g to 25 g of soy protein. This translates to two to four servings of soy nuts or soy milk. Women at high risk or who are being treated for breast, ovarian or uterine cancer should discuss their soy intake with their doctors—it can affect hormone levels that can fuel these cancers.

Sip Red Wine

Too much alcohol increases risk for high blood pressure—as well as heart disease and stroke. In moderation, however, red wine relaxes arteries and reduces risk for diabetes, a condition that often increases blood pressure. White wine and other forms of alcohol also reduce blood pressure, but red wine is a better choice because it contains more heart-protecting antioxidants known as flavonoids.

You'll get significant flavonoids from wines with a deep red color, such as cabernets. Specifically, grapevines that face harsher sun exposure and nutrient deprivation produce more flavonoids—cabernet sauvignon tops the list.

Red wine also is high in resveratrol, another antioxidant. One glass of red wine contains enough resveratrol to stimulate the body's production of nitric oxide. Pinot noir wine has more resveratrol than other types.

Recommended daily limit for red wine: No more than two glasses for men or one glass for women.

For people who can't drink alcohol, purple grape juice has some flavonoids and resveratrol but doesn't contain the full benefit provided by red wine.

More blood pressure–friendly foods…

•**Celery.** Celery is a centuries-old traditional Chinese medicine treatment for high

Slow Breathing Lowers Blood Pressure

You've probably heard that yoga, meditation and other forms of relaxation can reduce blood pressure.

An even simpler solution: Merely breathing more slowly, for just a few minutes a day, can do the same thing—and research shows that for some people, combining slow breathing with relaxation techniques can be as effective as drug therapy.

What to do: Once a day, take a little time to slow your breathing. Breathe in deeply for 10 seconds, then breathe out at the same rate. Repeat the cycle for 15 minutes.

Or try Resperate, an electronic breathing device that helps you synchronize your breathing ($300, Resperate.com).

Janet Bond Brill, PhD, RD, a registered dietitian and a nationally recognized expert in nutrition and cardiovascular disease prevention. She is the author of *Blood Pressure Down: The 10-Step Plan to Lower Your Blood Pressure in 4 Weeks Without Prescription Drugs.* DrJanet.com.

blood pressure, and various contemporary research studies affirm its benefit. Besides being rich in potassium, celery also contains 3-n-butyl phthalide, a compound that allows better blood flow by relaxing muscles in the walls of blood vessels.

•**Garlic.** A review article in the *Journal of Clinical Hypertension* called garlic "an agent with some evidence of benefit" in reducing high blood pressure, with some estimates saying that it can reduce blood pressure by 2%. Garlic contains the vasodilator and muscle-relaxing compound adenosine.

•**Beet juice.** Beets contain abundant nitrates, helpful in controlling blood pressure. Research from the Queen Mary University of London found that high blood pressure returned to normal levels when subjects were given two cups of beet juice per day.

•**Brown rice.** Recent research has shown that compounds in brown rice protect against hypertension by blocking an enzyme (angiotensin II) that increases blood pressure.

Eat Your Way to Low Cholesterol

Kenneth H. Cooper, MD, MPH, founder of the Cooper Clinic and The Cooper Institute for Aerobics Research, both in Dallas. A leading expert on preventive medicine and the health benefits of exercise, he is author of *Controlling Cholesterol the Natural Way.* The "Father of Aerobics," CooperAerobics.com

I f you have high cholesterol, your primary objective should be to find a way to lower it without drugs and their side effects. The good news is that just eating the right foods often can reduce cholesterol by 50 points or more.

Most people know to eat a low-fat diet, but there are certain foods that can help lower cholesterol that may surprise you…

Macadamia Nuts

Macadamia nuts are among the fattiest plant foods on the planet, about 76% total fat by weight. However, nearly all of the fat is monounsaturated. This type of fat is ideal because it lowers LDL (bad) cholesterol without depressing HDL (good) cholesterol.

A team at Hawaii University found that study participants who added macadamia nuts to their diets for just one month had total cholesterol levels of 191 milligrams/deciliter (mg/dL), compared with those eating the typical American diet (201 mg/dL). The greatest effect was on LDL cholesterol.

Macadamia nuts are higher than other nuts in monounsaturated fat, but all nuts are high in vitamin E, omega-3 fatty acids and other antioxidants. Data from the Harvard Nurses' Health Study found that people who ate at least five ounces of any kind of nut weekly were 35% less likely to suffer heart attacks than those who ate less than one ounce per month.

Caution: Moderation is important because nuts—macadamia nuts, in particular—are high in calories. Limit servings to between one and two ounces daily—about a small handful a day.

Rhubarb

Rhubarb is ideal for both digestive health and lowering cholesterol because it contains a mix of soluble (see "Oats" later in this article) and insoluble fibers.

A study reported in *Journal of the American College of Nutrition* found that participants who ate a little less than three ounces of rhubarb daily for four weeks had an average drop in LDL cholesterol of 9%.

This tart-tasting vegetable isn't only an ingredient in pies. You can cut and simmer the stalks and serve rhubarb as a nutritious side dish (add some low-calorie strawberry jam for a touch of sweetness).

Rice Bran

It's not as well known for lowering cholesterol as oats and oat bran, but rice bran is just about as effective and some people enjoy it more. A six-week study at University of California, Davis Medical Center found that people who ate three ounces daily of a product with rice bran had drops in total cholesterol of 8.3% and a reduction in LDL of 13.7%.

You can buy rice bran in most supermarkets—it's prepared like oatmeal. Or you can try prepared rice-bran breakfast cereals, such as Quaker Rice Bran Cereal and Kenmei Rice Bran.

Red Yeast Rice

Made from a yeast that grows on rice, red yeast rice contains monacolins, compounds that inhibit the body's production of cholesterol.

One study found that people who took red yeast rice supplements and did nothing else had drops in LDL of 23%. When the supplements were combined with healthy lifestyle changes, their LDL dropped by about 42%.

Red yeast rice may be less likely than statins to cause the side effect myopathy (a painful muscle disease).

Recommended dose: 600 milligrams (mg), twice daily. It is available online and at health-food stores.

Green Tea

Green tea is a concentrated source of polyphenols, which are among the most potent antioxidants. It can lower LDL cholesterol and prevent it from turning into plaque deposits in blood vessels. In one study, men who drank five cups of green tea daily had total cholesterol levels that were nine points lower than men who didn't drink green tea.

Three to five cups daily are probably optimal. Black tea also contains polyphenols but in lower concentrations than green tea.

Vitamins C and E

These vitamins help prevent cholesterol in the blood from oxidizing. Oxidized cholesterol is more likely to cling to artery walls and promote the development of atherosclerosis, the cause of most heart attacks.

I advise patients with high cholesterol to take at least 400 international units (IU) of d-alpha-tocopherol, the natural form of vitamin E, daily. You might need more if you engage in activities that increase oxidation, such as smoking.

For vitamin C, take 1,000 mg daily. People who get the most vitamin C are from 25% to 50% less likely to die from cardiovascular disease than those who get smaller amounts.

The Big Three

In addition to the above, some foods have long been known to reduce cholesterol, but they are so helpful that they bear repeating again...

•**Cholesterol-lowering margarines.** I use Benecol every day. It's a margarine that contains stanol esters, cholesterol-lowering compounds that are extracted from plants such as soy and pine trees. About 30 grams (g) of Benecol (the equivalent of about three to four pats of butter) daily will lower LDL by about 14%.

Similar products, such as Promise Buttery Spread, contain sterol esters. Like stanols, they help block the passage of cholesterol from the digestive tract into the bloodstream. We used to think that sterols weren't as effective as stanols for lowering cholesterol, but they appear to have comparable benefits.

•**Oats.** They are among the most potent nutraceuticals, natural foods with medicine-like properties. Both oat bran and oatmeal are high in soluble fiber. This type of fiber dissolves and forms a gel-like material in the intestine. The gel binds to cholesterol molecules, which prevents them from entering the bloodstream. A Harvard study that analyzed the results of 67 scientific trials found that even a small amount of soluble fiber daily lowered total cholesterol by five points. People who eat a total of 7 g to 8 g of soluble fiber daily typically see drops of up to 10%. One and a half cups of cooked oatmeal provides 6 g of fiber. If you don't like oatmeal, try homemade oat bran muffins. Soluble fiber also is found in such foods as kidney beans, apples, pears, barley and prunes.

Also helpful: Psyllium, a grain that's used in some breakfast cereals, such as Kellogg's All-Bran Bran Buds, and in products such as Metamucil. As little as 3 g to 4 g of psyllium daily can lower LDL by up to 20%.

•**Fish.** People who eat two to three servings of fish a week will have significant drops in both LDL and triglycerides, another marker for cardiac risk. One large study found that people who ate fish as little as once a week reduced their risk for a sudden, fatal heart attack by 52%.

I eat salmon, tuna, herring and sardines. Other good sources of omega-3 fatty acids include walnuts, ground flaxseed, tofu and canola oil.

Fish-oil supplements may provide similar protection, but they are not as effective as the natural food, which contains other beneficial nutrients as well.

Stop a Heart Attack Before It Happens

John A. Elefteriades, MD, the William W.L. Glenn Professor of Surgery and director of the Aortic Institute at Yale University and Yale–New Haven Hospital. He serves on the editorial boards of *The American Journal of Cardiology,* the *Journal of Cardiac Surgery, Cardiology* and *The Journal of Thoracic and Cardiovascular Surgery* and is the author of several books, including *Your Heart: An Owner's Guide.* HeartAuthorMD.com

Chest pain…shortness of breath…feeling faint…and/or discomfort in the arm—or even the neck, jaw or back. If you are overcome by such symptoms and perhaps even have an intense and sudden "sense of doom," you're likely to suspect a heart attack and rush to a hospital.

But wouldn't it be better to get a heads-up beforehand that a heart attack is on the way?

What most people don't realize: For about 60% of heart attack victims, warning symptoms do occur days or even weeks before the actual heart attack. But all too often, these signs are missed or shrugged off as something trivial.

What's behind this early-warning system? The blockage that creates a heart attack often develops over time and its symptoms, though they may be mild and elusive, should not be ignored.

Knowing the early red flags—including those you might not immediately connect to a heart problem—can allow you to see a doctor before a life-threatening heart attack occurs. Women, especially, can have symptoms that do not immediately bring heart disease to mind.

Important: If these symptoms are extreme and last for more than a few minutes—especially if they are accompanied by any of the more typical symptoms such as those described above—call 911. You could be having an actual heart attack. Even if these symptoms are mild to moderate but seem unexplained, call your doctor. If he/she cannot be reached but you're still concerned, go to the emergency room.

The following are examples of the subtle symptoms that can precede a heart attack—sometimes by days or weeks...

●**Fatigue.** If you feel more tired than usual, it's easy to tell yourself you're just growing older or getting out of shape. But pay attention! It could be the early-warning sign of heart trouble.

If your usual daily activities, whether it's walking the dog or cleaning the house, leave you feeling more tired than normal, talk to your doctor.

●**Flulike symptoms.** If you get hit with extreme fatigue, as well as weakness and/or feelings of light-headedness, you may think

---

Women, Pay Attention!

After a woman goes through menopause—when the body's production of heart-protective estrogen declines—her risk for a heart attack dramatically increases.

Important facts for women: More women die of heart disease each year than men. Nearly two-thirds of women who died from heart attacks had no history of chest pain. The higher death rate for women is likely due to the fact that women don't seek medical attention as promptly as men because they are afraid of being embarrassed if the symptoms turn out to be nothing serious. Don't let this fear stop you from seeking immediate care. If the symptoms turn out to be nothing serious, the emergency medical team will be happy!

What to watch for: While most (but not all) men experience crushing or squeezing chest pain (usually under the breastbone), women are more likely to have no chest pain (or simply a feeling of "fullness" in the chest). Also, women are more likely than men to suffer dizziness, shortness of breath and/or nausea as the main symptoms of heart attack. Most women (71%) experience sudden onset of extreme weakness that feels like the flu.

—John A. Elefteriades, MD

you're coming down with the flu. But people report having these same symptoms prior to a heart attack.

Call your doctor if you experience flulike symptoms but no fever (a telltale flu symptom).

Another clue: The flu generally comes on quickly, while flulike symptoms associated with heart disease may develop gradually.

•**Nausea and/or indigestion.** These are among the most overlooked symptoms of a heart attack—perhaps because they are typically due to gastrointestinal problems.

But if you are feeling sick to your stomach and throwing up, it could be a heart attack rather than food poisoning or some other stomach problem—especially if you're also sweating and your skin has turned an ashen color. If indigestion comes and goes, does not occur after a meal or doesn't improve within a day or so—especially if you're using antacids or antinausea medication—this could also mean heart problems. See a doctor.

•**Excessive perspiration.** If you are sweating more than usual—especially during times when you're not exerting yourself—it could mean that there are blockages. This can cause your heart to work harder, which may lead to excessive sweating. See your doctor. Clammy skin and night sweats also can be warning signs. This is likely to be a cold sweat, instead of the heat experienced in menopausal hot flashes. If sweating occurs with any of the classic heart attack symptoms described above, don't think twice—call 911.

•**Shortness of breath.** If you notice that you are beginning to feel more winded than usual, see your doctor. Shortness of breath can be a precursor to heart attack. If shortness of breath becomes stronger or lasts longer than usual, call 911. Shortness of breath may be your only symptom of a heart attack and may occur while you are resting or doing only minor physical activity.

•**Sexual dysfunction.** Men with heart problems that can lead to heart attack often have trouble achieving and/or keeping an erection. Because poor blood flow to the penis can be a sign of possible blockages elsewhere in the body, including the heart, erectile dysfunction can be an early-warning sign to get checked for cardiovascular disease. Men should absolutely discuss this symptom with their doctors.

Stroke: You Can Do Much More to Protect Yourself

Ralph L. Sacco, MD, chairman of neurology, the Olemberg Family Chair in Neurological Disorders and the Miller Professor of Neurology, Epidemiology and Public Health, Human Genetics and Neurosurgery at the Miller School of Medicine at the University of Miami.

N o one likes to think about having a stroke. But maybe you should.
  The grim reality: Stroke strikes about 800,000 Americans each year and is the leading cause of disability.

Now for the remarkable part: About 80% of strokes can be prevented. You may think that you've heard it all when it comes to preventing strokes—it's about controlling your blood pressure, eating a good diet and getting some exercise, right? *Actually, that's only part of what you can be doing to protect yourself…*

•**Even "low" high blood pressure is a red flag.** High blood pressure—a reading of 140/90 mmHg or higher—is widely known to increase one's odds of having a stroke. But even slight elevations in blood pressure may also be a problem.

An important recent study that looked at data from more than half a million patients found that those with blood pressure readings that were just slightly higher than a normal reading of 120/80 mmHg were more likely to have a stroke.

Dietary Fiber Cuts Stroke Risk

For every 7 grams (g) of fiber daily, the risk for a first-time stroke decreased by 7%, in a recent analysis. One serving of whole-wheat pasta or two servings of fruits and vegetables contain about 7 g of fiber. Other top fiber sources include brown rice, spelt, quinoa and other whole-grain foods…almonds and other nuts… lentils and other dried beans.

Recommended daily fiber intake: People age 50 or younger, 38 g (men) and 25 g (women)…over age 50, 30 g (men) and 21 g (women).

Victoria J. Burley, PhD, senior lecturer in nutritional epidemiology at University of Leeds, England, and coauthor of an analysis of eight studies, published in *Stroke*.

Any increase in blood pressure is worrisome. In fact, the risk for a stroke or heart attack doubles for each 20-point rise in systolic (the top number) pressure above 115/75 mmHg—and for each 10-point rise in diastolic (the bottom number) pressure.

My advice: Don't wait for your doctor to recommend treatment if your blood pressure is even a few points higher than normal. Tell him/her that you are concerned. Lifestyle changes—such as getting adequate exercise, avoiding excess alcohol and maintaining a healthful diet—often reverse slightly elevated blood pressure. Blood pressure consistently above 140/90 mmHg generally requires medication.

•**Sleep can be dangerous.** People who are sleep deprived—generally defined as getting less than six hours of sleep per night—are at increased risk for stroke.

What most people don't realize is that getting too much sleep is also a problem. When researchers at the University of Cambridge tracked the sleep habits of nearly 10,000 people over a 10-year period, they found that those who slept more than eight hours a night were 46% more likely to have a stroke than those who slept six to eight hours.

It is possible that people who spend less/more time sleeping have other, unrecognized conditions that affect both sleep and stroke risk.

Example: Sleep apnea, a breathing disorder that interferes with sleep, causes an increase in blood pressure that can lead to stroke. Meanwhile, sleeping too much can be a symptom of depression—another stroke risk factor.

My advice: See a doctor if you tend to wake up unrefreshed…are a loud snorer…or often snort or thrash while you sleep. You may have sleep apnea. If you sleep too much, also talk to your doctor to see if you are suffering from depression or some other condition that may increase your stroke risk.

What's the sweet spot for nightly shut-eye? When it comes to stroke risk, it's six to eight hours per night.

•**What you drink matters, too.** A Mediterranean-style diet—plenty of whole grains, legumes, nuts, fish, produce and olive oil—is perhaps the best diet going when it comes to minimizing stroke risk. A recent study concluded that about 30% of strokes could be prevented if people simply switched to this diet.

But there's more you can do. Research has found that people who drank six cups of green or black tea a day were 42% less likely to have strokes than people who did not drink tea. With three daily cups, risk dropped by 21%. The antioxidant epigallocatechin gallate or the amino acid L-theanine may be responsible.

•**Emotional stress shouldn't be pooh-poohed.** If you're prone to angry outbursts, don't assume it's no big deal. Emotional stress triggers the release of cortisol, adrenaline and other so-called stress hormones that can increase blood pressure and heart rate, leading to stroke.

In one study, about 30% of stroke patients had heightened negative emotions (such as anger) in the two hours preceding the stroke.

My advice: Don't ignore your mental health—especially anger (it's often a sign of depression, a potent stroke risk factor). If you're suffering from "nega-

Yogurt for Heart Health

In a review of data on 74,000 men and women with high blood pressure over 18 to 30 years, those who ate at least two weekly servings of yogurt had about a 20% lower risk for cardiovascular disease, including stroke, than those who consumed less than one serving of yogurt a month.

Theory: Yogurt, a fermented dairy product, reduces arterial stiffness.

Caution: Some yogurts contain added sugar, so opt for plain and add fruit or a drizzle of honey.

Justin Buendia, PhD, nutrition scientist and public health epidemiologist, Texas Department of State Health Services, Austin.

tive" emotions, exercise regularly, try relaxation strategies (such as meditation) and don't hesitate to get professional help.

•**Be alert for subtle signs of stroke.** The acronym "FAST" helps people identify signs of stroke. "F" stands for facial drooping—does one side of the face droop or is it numb? Is the person's smile uneven? "A" stands for arm weakness—ask the person to raise both arms. Does one arm drift downward? "S" stands for speech difficulty—is speech slurred? Is the person unable to speak or hard to understand? Can he/she repeat a simple sentence such as, "The sky is blue" correctly? "T" stands for time—if a person shows any of these symptoms (even if they go away), call 911 immediately. Note the time so that you know when symptoms first appeared.

But stroke can also cause one symptom that isn't widely known—a loss of touch sensation. This can occur if a stroke causes injury to the parts of the brain that detect touch. If you suddenly can't "feel" your fingers or toes—or have trouble with simple tasks such as buttoning a shirt—you could be having a stroke.

It's never normal to lose your sense of touch for an unknown reason—or to have unexpected difficulty seeing, hearing and/or speaking. Get to an emergency room!

Also important: If you think you're having a stroke, don't waste time calling your regular doctor. Call an ambulance, and ask to be taken to the nearest hospital with a primary stroke center. You'll get much better care than you would at a regular hospital emergency room.

A meta-analysis found that there were 21% fewer deaths among patients treated at stroke centers, and the surviving patients had faster recoveries and fewer stroke-related complications.

My advice: If you have any stroke risk factors, including high blood pressure, diabetes or elevated cholesterol, find out now which hospitals in your area have stroke centers. To find one near you, go to Hospital Maps.heart.org.

Be Vigilant About These Stroke Risk Factors

Louis R. Caplan, MD, senior neurologist at Beth Israel Deaconess Medical Center and a professor of neurology at Harvard Medical School, both in Boston. He has written or edited more than 40 books, including *Stroke (What Do I Do Now?)* and most recently *Navigating the Complexities of Stroke.*

What if there were more to preventing a stroke than keeping your blood pressure under control…getting regular exercise…watching your body weight…and not smoking? Researchers are now discovering that there is.

New thinking: While most stroke sufferers say that "it just came out of the blue," an increasing body of evidence shows that these potentially devastating "brain attacks" can be caused by conditions that you might ordinarily think are completely unrelated. Once you're aware of these "hidden" risk factors—and take the necessary steps to prevent or control them—you can improve your odds of never having a stroke. Recently discovered stroke risk factors…

Inflammatory Bowel Disease

Both Crohn's disease and ulcerative colitis can severely damage the large or small intestine. But that is not the only risk. Among patients who have either one of these conditions, known as inflammatory bowel disease (IBD), stroke is the third most common cause of death, according to some estimates.

During flare-ups, patients with IBD have elevated blood levels of substances that trigger clots—the cause of most strokes. A Harvard study, for example, found that many IBD patients have high levels of C-reactive protein (CRP), an inflammatory marker that has been linked to atherosclerotic lesions, damaged areas in blood vessels that can lead to stroke-causing clots in the brain.

If you have IBD: Ask your doctor what you can do to reduce your risk for blood clots and inflammation. Some patients with IBD can't take aspirin or other anticlotting drugs because these medications frequently cause in-

Stroke Fighter: Red Peppers

Eating red peppers and other vitamin C–rich fruits and veggies may reduce your risk for intracerebral hemorrhagic stroke (a blood vessel rupture in the brain). And what's so great about red peppers? At 190 mg per cup, they contain three times more vitamin C than an orange. Other good sources of vitamin C—broccoli and strawberries. Researchers believe that this vitamin may reduce stroke risk by regulating blood pressure and strengthening collagen, which promotes healthy blood vessels.

Stéphane Vannier, MD, neurologist, Pontchaillou University Hospital, Rennes, France, from research being presented at the annual meeting of the American Academy of Neurology.

testinal bleeding. Instead of aspirin, you might be advised to take an autoimmune medication such as *azathioprine* (Azasan, Imuran), which suppresses the immune system and reduces inflammation. During flare-ups, some patients are given steroids to further reduce inflammation.

Side effects, including nausea and vomiting with azathioprine use and weight gain and increased blood pressure with steroid use, usually can be minimized by taking the lowest possible dose.

Some physicians recommend omega-3 fish oil supplements for IBD, which are less likely to cause side effects. Ask your doctor whether these supplements (and what dose) are right for you.

Important: Strokes tend to occur in IBD patients when inflammation is most severe. To check inflammatory markers, CRP levels and erythrocyte sedimentation rate (ESR) can be measured. Tests for clotting include fibrinogen and d-dimer. The results of these tests will help determine the course of the patient's IBD treatment.

Migraines

Migraine headaches accompanied by auras (characterized by the appearance of flashing lights or other visual disturbances) are actually a greater risk factor for stroke than obesity, smoking or diabetes (see below), according to a startling study recently presented at the American Academy of Neurology's annual meeting.

When researchers use MRIs to examine blood vessels in the brain, they find more tiny areas of arterial damage in patients who have migraines with auras than in those who don't get migraines. (Research shows that there is no link between stroke and migraines that aren't accompanied by auras.)

If you have migraines with auras: Reduce your risk by controlling other stroke risk factors—don't smoke…lose weight if you're overweight…and control cholesterol levels.

Also: Women under age 50 who have migraines (with or without auras) may be advised to not use combined-hormone forms of birth control pills—they slightly increase risk for stroke. In addition, patients who have migraines with auras should not take beta-blockers, such as *propranolol* (Inderal), or the triptan drugs, such as *sumatriptan* (Imitrex), commonly used for migraine headaches. These drugs can also increase stroke risk. For frequent migraines with auras, I often prescribe the blood pressure drug *verapamil* (Calan) and a daily 325-mg aspirin. Ask your doctor for advice.

Rheumatoid Arthritis

Rheumatoid arthritis, unlike the common "wear-and-tear" variety (osteoarthritis), is an autoimmune disease that not only causes inflammation in the joints but may also trigger it in the heart, blood vessels and other parts of the body.

Arterial inflammation increases the risk for blood clots, heart attack and stroke. In fact, patients with severe rheumatoid arthritis were almost twice as likely to have a stroke as those without the disease, according to a study published in *Arthritis Care & Research*.

If you have rheumatoid arthritis: Work with your rheumatologist to manage flare-ups and reduce systemic inflammation. Your doctor will probably recommend that you take one or more anti-inflammatory painkillers, such as *ibuprofen* (Motrin). In addition, he/she might prescribe a disease-modifying antirheumatic drug (DMARD), such as *methotrexate* (Trexall), to slow the progression of the disease—and the increased risk for stroke. Fish oil also may be prescribed to reduce joint tenderness.

Strokes tend to occur in rheumatoid arthritis patients when inflammation is peaking. Ask your doctor if you should have the inflammation tests (CRP and ESR) mentioned in the IBD section.

Diabetes

If you have diabetes or diabetes risk factors—such as obesity, a sedentary lifestyle or a family history of diabetes—protect yourself. People with diabetes are up to four times more likely to have a stroke than those without it.

High blood sugar in people with diabetes damages blood vessels throughout the body, including in the brain. The damage can lead to both ischemic (clot-related) and hemorrhagic (bleeding) strokes.

If you have diabetes: Work closely with your doctor. Patients who achieve good glucose control with oral medications and/or insulin are much less likely to suffer from vascular damage.

Also important: Lose weight if you need to. Weight loss combined with exercise helps your body metabolize blood sugar more efficiently. In those with mild diabetes, weight loss combined with exercise may restore normal blood sugar levels…and can reduce complications and the need for medications in those with more serious diabetes.

Clotting Disorders

Any condition that affects the blood's normal clotting functions can increase risk for stroke.

Examples: Thrombocytosis (excessive platelets in the blood)…an elevated hematocrit (higher-than-normal percentage of red blood cells)…or Factor V Leiden (an inherited tendency to form blood clots). Clotting tests (fibrinogen and d-dimer) are recommended for these disorders.

If you have a clotting disorder: Ask your doctor what you can do to protect yourself from stroke.

Example: If you have an elevated hematocrit, your doctor might advise you to drink more fluids.

This is particularly important for older adults, who tend to drink less later in the day because they don't want to get up at night to urinate. I recommend that these patients drink approximately 80 ounces of noncaffeine-containing fluids during the day, stopping by 7 pm. People who don't take in enough fluids can develop "thick" blood that impedes circulation—and increases the risk for clots.

CHAPTER 13

Live Cancer Free

Delicious Cancer-Fighting Foods

Alice G. Bender, MS, RDN, associate director for nutrition programs at the American Institute for Cancer Research (AICR), a nonprofit organization that analyzes research and educates the public on the links between diet, physical exercise, weight loss and the prevention of cancer. AICR.org

Researchers are continually investigating foods that may help prevent cancer. But which ones have the strongest evidence?

The American Institute for Cancer Research (AICR), a nonprofit group that keeps tabs on cancer and diet research, recently identified the following foods as being among those having the strongest scientific evidence for fighting cancer...*

Pumpkin

Under the hard rind, orange pumpkin flesh is rich in carotenoids such as beta-carotene, alpha-carotene, lutein and zeaxanthin. A high intake of foods containing carotenoids has been linked to a lower incidence of many cancers, including those of the esophagus, mouth and larynx. Scientists have recently uncovered another protective compound in pumpkins—cucurmosin, a protein that has been shown to slow the growth of pancreatic cancer cells.

Smart idea: Eat pumpkin (plain, canned pumpkin is a convenient option) and the seeds.

*The studies cited in this article are only a small portion of the research supporting these cancer-fighting foods. The AICR and its international panel of experts review a much larger spectrum of research.

What to do: Eat a handful of pumpkin seeds (store-bought are fine) daily as a snack. To prepare your own, rinse fresh seeds in water, air-dry, add a touch of oil and bake at 350°F for 10 to 20 minutes.

Grapefruit

Grapefruit is a rich source of dietary fiber and vitamin C. The pink and red varieties also contain carotenoids (such as beta-carotene and lycopene) that decrease the DNA damage that can lead to cancer.

Scientific evidence: Strong research shows that foods like grapefruit help reduce risk for colorectal cancer. Other evidence suggests that it reduces risk for such malignancies as those of the esophagus, mouth, lung and stomach.

Helpful: Put red or pink grapefruit slices in a green salad with avocado. The tart grapefruit and creamy avocado are delicious together—and the fat in the avocado boosts the absorption of lycopene.

Caution: Grapefruit contains furanocoumarins, compounds that block a liver enzyme that breaks down some medications. (More than 85 medications interact with grapefruit, including cholesterol-lowering statins.) If you're thinking about eating more grapefruit and currently take one or more medications, talk to your doctor first.

Apples

An apple a day is good for you—but two may be even better!

Scientific evidence: In a study published in the *European Journal of Cancer Prevention*, people who ate an apple a day had a 35% lower risk for colorectal cancer—and those who ate two or more apples had a 50% lower risk.

Apples are protective because they contain several anticancer nutrients (many of them found in the peel), including fiber, vitamin C and flavonoids such as quercetin and kaempferol—plant compounds that have stopped the growth of cancer in cellular and animal studies. Research does not specify any particular type of apple as being more protective, so enjoy your favorite variety.

A quick and easy apple dessert: Core an apple, stuff it with raisins and cinnamon, top the stuffing with one tablespoon of apple cider or water, cover the apple with waxed paper and microwave for two minutes.

Mushrooms (Used in a Surprising Way)

When it comes to preventing cancer with diet, it's not only what you eat—it's also what you don't eat.

Scientific evidence: The evidence is convincing that eating too much red meat is linked to colorectal cancer. The AICR recommends eating no more than 18 ounces a week of cooked red meat (such as beef, pork and lamb).

A cancer-fighting meal extender: An easy, delicious way to lower your intake of red meat is to replace some of it in recipes with mushrooms. They're a perfect meat extender, with a savory, meaty taste and texture.

What to do: In a recipe that uses ground meat, replace one-third to one-half of the meat with chopped or diced mushrooms.

In a recent study, people who substituted one cup of white button mushrooms a day for one cup of lean ground beef consumed 123 fewer daily calories and lost an average of seven pounds after one year.

If you're heavier than you should be, losing weight means decreasing cancer risk—the AICR estimates that 122,000 yearly cases of cancer could be prevented if Americans weren't overweight or obese.

Five Cancer Risks—Even Your Doctor May Not Know About

Lynne Eldridge, MD, former clinical preceptor at the University of Minnesota Medical School in Minneapolis. She is the author of *Avoiding Cancer One Day at a Time.*

If you don't have any of the well-known risk factors for cancer, including smoking, a family history of cancer or long-term exposure to a carcinogen such as asbestos, you may think that your risk for the disease is average or even less than average.

What you may not realize: Although most of the cancer predispositions (genetic, lifestyle and environmental factors that increase risk for the disease) are commonly known, there are several medical conditions that also can increase your risk.

Unfortunately, many primary-care physicians do not link these conditions to cancer. As a result, they fail to prescribe the tests and treatments that could keep cancer at bay or reduce the condition's cancer-causing potential. *Medical conditions that increase your risk for cancer…*

1. Diabetes. The high blood sugar levels that occur with type 2 diabetes predispose you to heart attack, stroke, nerve pain, blindness, kidney failure, a need for amputation—and cancer.

New research: For every 1% increase in HbA1c—a measurement of blood sugar levels over the previous three months—there is an 18% increase in the risk for cancer, according to a recent study published in *Current Diabetes Reports.*

Other current studies have linked type 2 diabetes to a 94% increased risk for pancreatic cancer…a 38% increased risk for colon cancer…a 15% to 20% higher risk for postmenopausal breast cancer…and a 20% higher risk or blood cancers such as non-Hodgkin's lymphoma and leukemia.

What to do: If you have type 2 diabetes, make sure your primary-care physician orders regular screening tests for cancer, such as colonoscopy and mammogram.

Screening for pancreatic cancer is not widely available, but some of the larger cancer centers (such as the H. Lee Moffitt Cancer Center & Research Institute in Tampa, Florida, and the Mayo Clinic in Rochester, Minnesota) offer it to high-risk individuals. This typically includes people with long-standing diabetes (more than 20 years) and/or a family history of pancreatic cancer. The test involves an ultrasound of both the stomach and small intestine, where telltale signs of pancreatic cancer can be detected.

Also work with your doctor to minimize the cancer-promoting effects of diabetes. For example, control blood sugar levels through a diet that emphasizes slow-digesting foods that don't create spikes in blood sugar levels, such as vegetables and beans…get regular exercise—for example, 30 minutes of walking five or six days a week…and consider medical interventions, such as use of the diabetes drug *metformin* (Glucophage).

2. Helicobacter pylori infection. This bacterial infection of the lining of the stomach can cause stomach inflammation (gastritis) and ulcers in the stomach or upper small intestine. It also causes most stomach cancers.

Startling statistic: An infection with H. pylori triggers a 10-fold increase in your predisposition to stomach cancer. Getting treatment for an H. pylori infection lowers your risk for stomach cancer by 35% but does not eliminate the risk—perhaps due to lingering inflammation. What's most important is to avoid other inflammation-causing habits such as smoking.

What to do: If you are diagnosed with gastritis or a stomach or intestinal ulcer, ask your doctor to check for an H. pylori infection—and to treat it with antibiotics if it is detected. Research shows that a fecal analysis is the most accurate way to detect H. pylori.

3. "Iron overload" disease. This hereditary condition (known technically as hemochromatosis) affects one out of every 200 people, causing them to absorb and store too much dietary iron—in the liver, heart, joints and pancreas. Hemochromatosis also increases a person's risk for cancer (particularly liver cancer).

New research: In a study of more than 8,000 people reported in the *Journal of Internal Medicine*, iron overload increased the risk for any cancer nearly fourfold.

Iron overload should be suspected if you have or had a relative (including a second-degree relative such as a grandparent) with the condition...you have a family history of early heart disease (beginning at age 50 or earlier)...you have a family history of cirrhosis without obvious reasons such as alcoholism or hepatitis...or you have the symptoms of hemochromatosis (joint pain, fatigue, abdominal pain and a bronze appearance to the skin).

What to do: Ask your doctor for a serum ferritin test. If the test confirms iron overload, your doctor can simply and quickly correct the problem with regular bloodletting—a pint of blood once or twice per week until iron levels return to normal, and then three to four times per year.

4. Inflammatory bowel disease (IBD). This autoimmune disease attacks the lining of the intestine, causing symptoms such as abdominal cramping and bloating, bloody diarrhea and urgent bowel movements. The disease takes two main forms—ulcerative colitis (affecting the colon) and Crohn's disease (usually affecting the small intestine). Both forms predispose you to colon cancer.

Recent research: People age 67 and older with ulcerative colitis have a 93% higher risk for colorectal cancer...people of the same age group with Crohn's disease have a 45% higher risk, according to a 2011 study reported in *Digestive Diseases and Sciences.*

Problem: IBD can come and go in flare-ups that occur only once every five to 10 years. This can lead your primary-care physician to underestimate the severity of the problem and your risk for colon cancer.

What to do: IBD usually is diagnosed between the ages of 15 and 30. If you have ulcerative colitis that involves the entire colon, you should have your first colonoscopy eight years after diagnosis or at the standard age of 50 (whichever comes first) and then have another every one to two years thereafter.

If you have ulcerative colitis that involves only the left colon (which represents a somewhat smaller cancer risk than when the entire colon is affected) or Crohn's disease, you should receive your first colonoscopy 12 to 15 years after your diagnosis or at age 50 and then another every one to two years thereafter.

5. Polyps detected in a relative. Most people think that a hereditary predisposition to colon cancer means that you have a first-degree relative (parent, sibling or child) who was diagnosed with the disease.

Surprising fact: If you have a first-degree relative who had a colonoscopy that detected an adenomatous polyp (adenoma)—a type of growth that can turn into cancer within two to five years—you also have a predisposition to colon cancer.

New research: Having a first-degree relative with an adenoma appears to make you four times more likely to develop colorectal cancer, according to a report in *Annals of Internal Medicine*.

What to do: Have a first colonoscopy 10 years earlier than the age at which your relative's adenoma was detected and repeat it every five to 10 years (depending on results). That should give plenty of time to detect (and remove) an adenoma so it can never turn into cancer.

Interesting: Some cancer centers also advise earlier screening if a second-degree relative, such as a grandparent, had colon cancer.

Secrets to Getting the Best Colonoscopy

Douglas K. Rex, MD, a Distinguished Professor of Medicine at Indiana University School of Medicine and director of endoscopy at Indiana University Hospital, both in Indianapolis. He is coauthor of the colorectal cancer screening recommendations of the American College of Gastroenterology as well as current chair of the US Multi-Society Task Force on Colorectal Cancer and coauthor of the recommendations on quality in colonoscopy for this group.

If you're age 50 or older, chances are you've had a colonoscopy—and maybe more than one. If so, you've taken a crucial step in protecting your health.

Why this test is so important: It's estimated that if every person age 50 and older had a colonoscopy, 64% of people with colorectal cancer would have never developed the disease.

But since you are going to the trouble to get this test (and we all know the bowel-cleansing prep is no picnic), then it also makes sense to make sure you're getting the best possible screening. *How to ensure that you get the maximum cancer protection from your colonoscopy…*

How Good Is Your Doctor?

One of the most important aspects of a colonoscopy is the doctor's ability to detect a type of polyp called an adenoma—the doctor's so-called "adenoma detection rate" (ADR). This varies widely depending on the doctor's skill.

If your doctor has a low ADR, you're more likely to get colon cancer before your next colonoscopy. Gastroenterologists are more likely to have good ADRs than primary-care physicians and general surgeons who might perform colonoscopies, but there's a wide range of performance within each group.

Precisely defined, a doctor's ADR is the percentage of screening colonoscopies in patients age 50 or older during which he/she detects one or more adenomas. My advice: Look for a doctor with an ADR of 20% or higher in women and 30% or higher in men (who have more adenomas)…or a "mixed-gender" rate of 25% or higher—in other words, the doctor detects at least one adenoma in 25% of the screening colonoscopies he conducts.

Startling recent finding: A 10-year study published in *The New England Journal of Medicine* evaluated more than 300,000 colonoscopies conducted by 136 gastroenterologists—and found that for every 1% increase in ADR, there was a 3% reduction in the risk of developing colorectal cancer before the next colonoscopy. This means that having your colonoscopy performed by a doctor with a high ADR (as described earlier) is a must for optimal screening. But how does a patient ask about his doctor's ADR without seeming to question the physician's competence?

My advice: Ask about your doctor's ADR on the phone, during the colonoscopy scheduling process, when you are talking to an administrator or a nurse. If that person doesn't know, request that someone get back to you with the number. That will make your query less confrontational.

However: Even your doctor may not know his own ADR. Monitoring of ADRs is endorsed by several professional medical societies, such as the American Society for Gastrointestinal Endoscopy and the American College of Gastroenterology, but there is no law mandating that doctors must track it. Or your doctor may refuse to disclose his ADR—a response you should find concerning. If you don't get the information you need from your doctor, it's probably a good idea to find a new one.

Also important: Make sure your colonoscopy is being performed with a high-definition colonoscope, the current state-of-the-art in colonoscopy. Inquire about this when you ask about a doctor's ADR.

A Better Bowel Prep

Another key to a truly preventive colonoscopy is the preparation. Before the procedure, a patient drinks a defecation-inducing liquid (prep) that cleanses the rectum and colon of stool so that the doctor can clearly see the lining. In some patients, a four-liter prep (about one gallon), or even more, is best for optimal cleansing. If you don't have a condition associated with slow bowel motility, such as chronic constipation, or use constipating medications such as opioids, you may be eligible for one of the regimens that requires only two or three liters of fluid. (A pill preparation is also available, but it is seldom used because it can cause kidney damage.) Ask your doctor what regimen will give you the best combination of excellent cleansing and tolerability.

A common mistake: Many people think that they can drink the prep one to two days before the procedure and then drink nothing but clear fluids (such as Gatorade, apple juice or water) until the day of the colonoscopy.

But even during the prep, the small intestine (the section of bowel after the stomach and before the colon) continues to produce chyme, a thick, mucousy secretion that sticks to the walls of the ascending colon—so that seven to eight hours after drinking the prep the colon is no longer completely clean.

Best: A split prep, with half the prep ingested the day before the procedure and half ingested four to five hours before (the middle of the night when the colonoscopy is scheduled for the morning...or the morning when the colonoscopy is scheduled for the afternoon). Scientific evidence: Split preparation improves ADR by 26%, according to a study in *Gastrointestinal Endoscopy.*

Also helpful: Drinking the prep can be difficult, even nauseating. How to make it more palatable...

Chill the liquid thoroughly, and drink it with a straw. Follow each swallow with ginger ale or another good-tasting clear liquid. Suck on a clear menthol lozenge after you drink the prep. And if you throw up the prep, wait 30 minutes (until you feel less nauseated) and then continue drinking the prep as instructed—it can still work.

Several recent studies have found that eating a fiber-free diet all or part of the day prior to colonoscopy allows for better cleansing of the colon. Some doctors advise avoiding high-fiber foods such as corn, seeds and nuts for about a week before a colonoscopy. Ask your doctor what he advises for you.

Deadly Melanoma: Best Prevention, Detection and Treatment Breakthroughs

The late **Albert Lefkovits, MD,** an associate clinical professor of dermatology at Mount Sinai School of Medicine and codirector of the Mount Sinai Dermatological Cosmetic Surgery Program, both in New York City.

Melanoma is the most dangerous form of skin cancer. It's particularly frightening because it's more likely than other cancers to spread (metastasize) to other parts of the body. More than 76,000 Americans are diagnosed with melanoma each year, and between 8,000 and 9,000 will die from it.

Good news: New technology increases the chances that a melanoma will be detected early—and when it is, you have a 95% to 97% chance of surviving. The prognosis is worse after the disease has spread. However, therapy has been revolutionized to extend survival times, particularly in the last two years.

Who's at Risk?

A study published in *Journal of Investigative Dermatology* found that melanoma rates increased by 3.1% annually between 1992 and 2004—and the incidence continues to rise.

The increase is due to several reasons. The US population is aging, and older adults are more likely to get melanoma (though it is a leading cause of cancer death in young adults). Public-awareness campaigns have increased the rate of cancer screenings (though officials would like the screening rates to be even higher), and more screenings mean an increase in melanoma diagnoses.

If you are a fair-skinned Caucasian, your lifetime risk of getting melanoma is about one in 50. The risk is lower among African Americans, Hispanics (although over the past decade incidence has increased 20% among Hispanics) and Asians, but they're more likely to die from it.

Reason: They often develop cancers on "hidden" areas (such as the soles of the feet), where skin changes aren't readily apparent.

Important: Don't be complacent just because you avoid the sun or use sunscreen. Many cancers appear in areas that aren't exposed to the sun, such as between the toes or around the anus.

State-of-the-Art Screening

Melanomas grow slowly. Patients who get an annual skin checkup are more likely to get an early diagnosis than those who see a doctor only when a mole or skin change is clearly abnormal.

Doctors used to depend on their eyes (and sometimes a magnifying glass) to examine suspicious areas. But eyes-only examinations can identify melanomas only about 60% of the time.

Better: An exam called epiluminescence microscopy. The doctor takes photographs of large areas of skin. Then he/she uses a device that magnifies suspicious areas in the photos. The accuracy of detecting melanomas with this technique is about 90%.

The technology also allows doctors to look for particular changes, such as certain colors or a streaked or globular appearance, that indicate whether a skin change is malignant or benign. This can reduce unnecessary biopsies.

Few private-practice physicians can afford the equipment that's used for these exams. You might want to get your checkups at a medical center or dermatology practice that specializes in early melanoma detection. If this isn't possible, ask your doctor if he/she uses a handheld dermatoscope. It's a less expensive device that's still superior to the unaided eye.

Recent Treatments

In the last few years, the FDA has approved several medications for patients with late-stage melanoma. These drugs don't cure the disease but can help patients live longer.

•*Ipilimumab* (**Yervoy**) is a biologic medication, a type of synthetic antibody that blocks a cellular "switch" that turns off the body's ability to fight cancer. A study of 676 patients with late-stage melanoma found that those who took the drug survived, on average, for 10 months after starting treatment, compared with 6.4 months for those in a control group.

•*Vemurafenib* (**Zelboraf**) may double the survival time of patients with advanced melanoma. It works by targeting a mutation in the BRAF V600E gene, which is present in about 50% of melanoma patients. Researchers who conducted a study published in *The New England Journal of Medicine* found that more than half of patients who took the medication had at least a 30% reduction in tumor size. In about one-third of patients, the medication slowed or stopped the progression of the cancer.

•**Combination treatment.** Each of these medications attacks tumors in different ways. They can be used in tandem for better results. Drugs such as Yervoy and two additional newly approved drugs, *nivolumab* (Opdivo) and *pembrolizumab* (Keytruda), have been shown to work in combination with each other, affording much more effective therapy and giving new hope to melanoma patients. Also, new developments in vaccine therapy offer promise for the future, but are not FDA-approved at this time.

Both drugs can have serious side effects. For now, they're recommended only for a select group of patients.

Self-Protection

Take steps to protect yourself…

•**Check your skin monthly.** It's been estimated that deaths from melanoma could be reduced by 60% if everyone would do a monthly skin exam to look for suspicious changes. Look for asymmetric moles in which one part is distinctly different from the other part…moles with an irregular border…color variations…a diameter greater than 6 millimeters (mm), about one-quarter inch…or changes in appearance over time.

•**Get a yearly checkup with a dermatologist.** It's nearly impossible to self-inspect all of the areas on your body where melanoma can appear. I advise patients to see a dermatologist every year for full-body mapping. The doctor will make a note (or photograph) of every suspicious area and track the areas over time.

Important: New moles rarely appear in people over the age of 40. A mole that appears in patients 40 years and older is assumed to be cancer until tests show otherwise.

•**Use a lot of sunscreen.** Even though melanoma isn't caused only by sun exposure, don't get careless. Apply a sunscreen with an SPF of at least 30 whenever you go outdoors. Use a lot of sunscreen—it takes about two ounces of sunscreen (about the amount in a shot glass) to protect against skin cancer. Reapply it about every two hours or immediately after getting out of the water.

•**Don't use tanning salons.** Researchers who published a study in *Journal of the National Cancer Institute* found that people who got their tans at tanning salons—that use tanning lamps and tanning beds that emit UV radiation—at least once a month were 55% more likely to develop a malignant melanoma than those who didn't artificially tan.

CHAPTER 14

Mind and Body

Loneliness Harms Your Health

Gregory T. Eells, PhD, associate director of Gannett Health Services and director of Counseling and Psychological Services at Cornell University in Ithaca, New York. Dr. Eells is also a past president of the Association for University and College Counseling Center Directors.

Oh, those long, lonesome days…and nights! Most of us occasionally feel that way. But what if you are lonely more often than not? Plenty of people are.

Important new finding: Persistent loneliness is being linked to a growing list of health problems, including insomnia, cardiovascular disease and Alzheimer's disease. Even more startling is the fact that loneliness raises the risk for premature death among adults age 50 and older by 14%.

So for the sake of your health—and happiness—here's what you need to know about loneliness…

Are You Lonely?

While it's easy to assume that anyone who is struggling with loneliness would know that he/she is lonely, that's often not the case. For many people, that extreme sense of social disconnection—the feeling that no one really knows you and what your life is like—is so familiar and constant that they don't even realize that they're lonely. And friends and family might not necessarily recognize that a friend or loved one is lonely.

Of course, most of us do need some time by ourselves, and solitude—the opportunity to think and feel quietly without the distraction and demands of other people—is rightly valued. But loneliness is very different.

Here are some red flags that you may be lonely: You spend hours of alone time on the computer (perhaps surfing the Internet or following the activities of "friends" on social media sites)…you have pangs of anger or envy when others around you are happy…and/or you feel a vague sense of dissatisfaction even when you are spending time with other people.

But just as you can be alone without being lonely, you can be lonely without being alone. Someone who looks happy and well connected from the outside—the person who invites 20 of his/her closest friends to a party—may still feel empty and isolated inside. Nor are romantic relationships or marriage a surefire defense against loneliness. Feeling uncomfortably alone and alienated is a frequent complaint of troubled couples.

Why It's Bad For You

The connection between loneliness and depression has been established for quite some time. People who have depression often withdraw from social situations and have feelings of loneliness. But only recently have researchers discovered that loneliness itself is linked to elevated blood pressure, increased stress hormones and impaired immune function.

A new study has also found that the more lonely that people reported themselves to be, the more fragmented—and less restful—was their average night's sleep.

Loneliness also exacts a huge toll when people turn to unhealthy behaviors to avoid the pain it brings—if we don't try to drink it away, for example, then we might spend far too many hours at work to busy ourselves rather than face painful time alone.

How to Overcome Loneliness

Alleviating loneliness is like falling asleep or growing a garden—you can't force it to happen, but you can create conditions that encourage it to unfold. *Here's how…*

SECRET #1: **Share more about yourself.** Sharing the details of your life with others and showing vulnerability will foster deep connections and minimize loneliness. This may feel risky. After all, you might run up against rejection or disapproval, but such fears are usually groundless. Nothing ventured, nothing gained!

Example: You might ask a friend to have coffee and share with him/her discipline problems you are having with your teenage daughter.

SECRET #2: Make room for "small" connections. While quantity doesn't replace quality in relationships, momentary contacts do add to your sense of being part of the social world around you.

Exchange a few extra words with the clerk at your local convenience store, and smile at those you pass on the street. These pleasant interactions will prime you for deeper, more meaningful ones with close friends and family.

SECRET #3: Be part of something big. Meaningful activity will bring you in contact with like-minded others. OK, so maybe volunteering in a hospital or soup kitchen isn't your thing. Perhaps you would rather get involved with your local political party…tutor a child who is struggling in school… join a gardening club…or get involved at your house of worship.

Your local newspaper and websites such as Meetup.com and Groups.yahoo. com are great resources for finding local groups involved in a wide variety of activities that might interest you.

Show up for whatever new activity you choose for several weeks, and if you're not feeling more connected by the end of that time, then look for something else that might be more to your liking.

SECRET #4: Don't hole up by yourself when your life changes. For most people, significant changes such as job loss, the death of a loved one, divorce or retirement provide a good excuse to shut out others—and the perfect setup for loneliness. But don't let the natural tendency to withdraw at such times go on for more than a few months.

Challenge yourself to set up two outings a week with a friend, neighbor or family member to get yourself out of the house.

SECRET #5: Consider getting a pet. Pets are more than mere company… dogs, cats, birds and even guinea pigs are, after all, fellow creatures that have their own feelings and are often responsive to ours. These are real connections, too.

If you don't have the time to care for a pet full time, consider sharing a pet. There are several sites (CityDogShare.org) that enable you to meet people near you who are interested in doing this. Or volunteer at your local animal shelter.

Both of these activities are great ways to connect with animals and animal lovers.

Fight Depression Using Only Your Mind

Zindel Segal, PhD, CPsych, the Cameron Wilson Chair in Depression Studies at the University of Toronto, and head of the Cognitive Behavioural Therapy Unit at the Centre for Addiction and Mental Health, both in Toronto, Canada. He is a coauthor of *The Mindful Way through Depression: Freeing Yourself from Chronic Unhappiness.*

S uffering from depression is very different from being sad. Sadness is a normal part of life. Depression is a constellation of psychological and physical changes that persist, unrelenting, for a minimum of two weeks—and often much longer.

For those affected, depression often becomes an ongoing issue—those who have faced it once have a 40% chance of experiencing an episode in the future and those who already have had multiple episodes face up to an 80% chance of additional recurrences.

Depression is most commonly treated with medication that regulates the brain's chemistry and with professional counseling, which helps people take effective action in the face of the low motivation and pessimism that often define depression.

Exciting tool: In the last decade or so, a new technique has been shown in studies to help sufferers head off depression before it takes hold. The technique is called mindfulness—paying attention to the present moment, without judgment, in order to see things more clearly.

Life on Automatic Pilot

Mindfulness can prevent depression from taking hold of us because the alternative—our usual state—is that we operate on "automatic pilot." Our minds are elsewhere as we perform mundane activities.

Example: You're taking a shower, but wondering what's waiting in your e-mail.

If we let it, this automatic pilot also will select our moods and our emotional responses to events—and the responses it chooses can be problematic. For instance, if you make a minor misstep in some area of your life, your autopilot might select as your emotional response feelings of anger, failure and/or inadequacy, even though the event might have been completely inconsequential.

Because your mind is not paying full attention to the situation, you might not grasp that the negative feelings are greatly out of proportion to what's really going on. You only know that you feel bad. When these negative feelings persist, they can pull you into the downward spiral of depression.

Example: A friend mentions that one of the stocks in his portfolio has turned a profit. Your investments have not been as successful, and your autopilot selects inadequacy as your primary emotional response. This may sound like an overreaction, but in someone who is prone to depression, these feelings can expand into a full-blown episode.

Mindfulness can be an antidote to automatic pilot. By becoming more aware of the world around us, we experience life directly, not filtered through our minds' relentless ruminations. We learn to see events for what they are rather than what our autopilot might turn them into. That helps us to derail potential episodes of depression before they have a chance to take hold. It typically takes two weeks or longer for depression to fully sink in, so there is often plenty of time to stop the process.

Becoming Mindful

Learning to be mindful involves more than simply paying attention. You must reorient your senses so that you experience a situation with your whole mind and heart and with all of your senses.

Try it out: Pick up a raisin. Hold it, feel it, examine it as if you had never seen anything like it before. Explore the raisin's folds and texture. Watch the way light shines off of its skin. Inhale its aroma. Then gently place it on your tongue. Notice how your hand knows exactly where to put it. Explore the raisin in your mouth before biting. Then chew once or twice. Experience the waves of taste and the sensation of chewing. Notice how the taste and texture change as you chew. Once you swallow, try to feel the raisin moving through your digestive system.

Keep it up: Practice the following three steps every day to make mindfulness a regular part of your life—and episodes of depression less likely…

1. Focus on your breath. Focusing your attention on your breath is perhaps the simplest, most effective way to anchor your mind in the moment. You think only of this breath. You can do this anytime, anywhere.

Depressed? Give New Eyeglasses a Try

Eyeglasses ease depression among the elderly.

Recent finding: After two months, seniors who received properly prescribed eyeglasses had higher scores for activities, hobbies and social interaction—and fewer signs of depression—than seniors with similar visual acuity who were not given new eyeglasses.

Cynthia Owsley, PhD, professor, department of ophthalmology, University of Alabama at Birmingham, and leader of a study of 78 nursing home residents, published in *Archives of Ophthalmology*.

2. Watch your thoughts drift by like clouds. See them, acknowledge them, but do not attempt to reason them away. Some people attempt to use logic to escape depression. They tell themselves, My life is pretty good—I should be happy. This just leads to troubling questions like If my life is good, why am I so unhappy? What's wrong with me?

It is also tempting to try to push negative thoughts away so that you don't have to deal with them at all. Unfortunately, the thoughts are still there even if you refuse to acknowledge them.

Better: When you feel bad, reflect on what is bothering you. Try to uncover the original thought or event that set off your bad feelings. Then view it as just a thought, something independent from you even though it has popped into your head. Do not dismiss it, though. Even if the thought or the event that caused it was trivial, the feelings it has prompted are real and significant.

Next, notice any physical sensations that you are experiencing. Does your throat feel tight? Is your mouth dry? Are there butterflies in your stomach? Just as you are learning to watch your feelings float by, watch these physical sensations in a detached way. If you can learn to spot the onset of these sensations, you will be able to identify the early signs of depression sooner—and head off the bad feelings before they take root.

3. Take action.

Ask yourself: Does this thought have any merit? Is it connected to negative thoughts that I have had in the past? What can I do to make myself feel better about this issue?

Example: You feel depressed about your work life even though you are doing fine in your job. When you reflect on these negative thoughts, you realize that they began recently, when you learned that your brother received a promotion. You feel left behind because it has been some time since your last promotion.

What actions could you take to allay these negative feelings? Perhaps you could speak with your supervisor about your job performance and your prospects for future promotions...or contact a headhunter to remind yourself that you have other options.

With any problematic thought, identifying it quickly and taking some positive action is often enough to head off depression.

Important: Learning the mindfulness approach can be useful for preventing future bouts of depression—not for combating an episode that is already under way. When people are in the midst of depression, they typically cannot concentrate sufficiently to practice mindfulness. It is better to use the technique between episodes of depression so that it becomes a natural part of your thought process.

Where to Find Help Against Depression

For information about depression and links to local support, contact...

- **National Institute of Mental Health,** 866-615-6464, NIMH.nih.gov.
- **National Alliance on Mental Illness,** 800-950-6264, NAMI.org.

Let Go of Toxic Memories

Thomas H. Crook III, PhD, CEO of Cognitive Research Corporation and a psychologist in private practice in St. Petersburg, Florida. He is author of numerous books, including *The Memory Advantage.* CogRes.com

A toxic memory turned constant companion is a harmful bad habit—and like any bad habit, it can be broken. *Steps...*

1. Select a favorite positive memory. You can choose an event that specifically contradicts your toxic memory (for instance, the day you learned to ski despite being a "hopeless klutz")...or choose a completely unrelated experience, such as your first date with your spouse.

2. Write down as many details as you can recall. Where did you go? What did you wear? Did you dance to a certain song or see a stunning sunset? How did that first kiss feel? Tap into all your senses.

3. Practice conjuring up this happy memory. Let this personal "movie" play inside your head during relaxed moments. Soon you'll be able to recall it vividly at will, even when stressed or depressed.

4. Mentally hit an "eject" button whenever a toxic memory pops into your head, replacing it with thoughts of the happy memory.

Fulfilling Emotional Needs

If the technique above isn't working, your toxic memory may be more than a bad habit—it may be fulfilling some unmet need. Ask yourself, "How am I benefiting by holding onto this painful memory?" This insight will help you explore more productive ways to meet that need, thus diminishing the power of the toxic memory. *Consider...*

●**Does thinking of yourself as unlucky let you avoid taking responsibility for your life?** On a sheet of paper, make two columns, labeled "good luck" and "bad luck," then list examples from your own life of each type of experience. You will see that your whole life hasn't been a series of misfortunes. Next, identify the role played by your own efforts—rather than good luck—in creating each positive experience...and give yourself due credit.

●**Is there a certain pleasure for you in resenting other people for past unpleasantness?** (Be honest with yourself!) Develop a habit of doing small favors that make people respond to you in a positive way. Smile at everyone you pass on the sidewalk, yield to other drivers trying to enter your lane, say a sincere "thank you" to a surly cashier. A conscious and voluntary decision to be of service to others can help you overcome old resentments, relegate toxic memories to the past and find pleasure in the here and now.

If you feel traumatized: After an extremely traumatic experience, it is normal to fixate on the event for a time. However, if you are seriously disturbed by recurrent memories of the trauma months or even years later, you may have post-traumatic stress disorder (PTSD). Symptoms include nightmares or obsessive mental reenactments of the event...frequent fear or anger...trouble concentrating...feelings of guilt, hopelessness or emotional numbness.

Defusing traumatic memories may require the help of a mental-health professional.

Recommended: Cognitive-behavioral therapy (CBT), which focuses on changing harmful thought patterns rather than on lengthy exploration of past experiences.

Referrals: National Association of Cognitive-Behavioral Therapists, NACBT. org. With CBT, even seriously toxic memories can become more manageable—and you can move on with your life.

Reconcile with Your Grief...and Live Happily Again

Alan D. Wolfelt, PhD, CT (certified thanatologist, which indicates an expertise in strategies for coping with death), founder and director of the Center for Loss and Life Transition in Fort Collins, Colorado. He is the author of several books, including *Understanding Your Grief* and *Healing a Spouse's Grieving Heart*. CenterforLoss.com

When someone you love dies, it's natural to feel the pain of your loss—and to grieve. But too many people try hard not to feel the pain. While it's understandable to want to avoid pain, it's a mistake to do so. People who appear to be "doing well" with their grief sometimes develop chronic, low-grade depression, anxiety and/or addiction to alcohol or drugs as they self-treat their emotional pain.

Recent developments: An increasing body of research is now also linking this type of unreconciled grief (meaning an inability to move forward in life without the person who died) to a wide range of physical ailments, including fatigue, headache, high blood pressure and heart disease.

For many people, grief is prolonged and unresolved because there are so many misconceptions surrounding it. Among the most common—and dangerous—misconceptions about grief...

MISCONCEPTION #1: Grief and mourning are the same thing. People tend to use the words "grieving" and "mourning" interchangeably, but they have different meanings.

Grief is the constellation of internal thoughts and feelings you have when someone you love dies. Mourning is when you take the grief you have on the inside and express it outside yourself.

Examples of mourning: Talking about the person who died. Crying. Expressing your thoughts and feelings through art or music. Celebrating anniversary dates that held meaning for the person who died.

Many people grieve but don't mourn. When you don't honor a loss by acknowledging it—first to yourself, and then to others—your grief will accumulate. The denied losses then come flowing out in other ways, such as depression and physical problems...all of which compound the pain of your loss.

MISCONCEPTION #2: You should move away from grief, not toward it. Our society does not give people much time to grieve. They're expected to get "back to normal" in short order.

This attitude leads many people to either grieve in isolation or attempt to run away from their grief through various means, such as overworking or abusing alcohol or drugs. Masking or moving away from your grief creates anxiety, confusion and depression.

What to do: Continually remind yourself that leaning toward—not away—from the pain will help you heal. To lean toward the pain, when you are feeling bad, stop and allow yourself to feel the emotion by talking to someone or writing about it.

MISCONCEPTION #3: **Grief is mainly about the physical loss of the person who died.** The death of a loved one creates many secondary losses—such as connections to yourself and the world around you.

Examples: You can lose the self ("I feel like a part of me died")...identity (such as your role as a spouse or child)...security (for example, a widow may not feel as safe in her home)...and meaning (when dreams for the future are shattered).

Important: Understanding the range and depth of your personal losses can help you be more self-compassionate. This involves showing sensitivity toward yourself for what you're going through.

Physical self-compassion can include eating well, exercising regularly and getting enough sleep.

Mental self-compassion can mean asking yourself two questions on a daily basis that will help you survive the difficult months of grieving and learn to love life again...

1. What do I want? (now that the person you love is gone). Ask yourself what's doable and what you'd like to accomplish today.

2. What is wanted of me? (Who depends on you? What skills and experience can you bring to others?)

Social self-compassion can include finding a grief "buddy"—a friend who has also had a loss—and/or joining a grief support group. To find a group near you, check with local hospices and funeral homes.

Grief forces us to consider what life is about and what greater purpose there might be for our lives. Spiritual self-compassion can mean starting each day with a meditation or spending time in nature.

MISCONCEPTION #4: **After a loved one dies, the goal should be to "get over" your grief as soon as possible.** Grief is not a problem that you can solve or an illness from which you recover. Rather, you become reconciled to your grief—you integrate the new reality of moving forward in life without the person who died. With reconciliation comes a renewed sense of energy and confidence, an ability to fully acknowledge the reality of the death and a capacity to become re-involved in the activities of living.

MISCONCEPTION #5: When grief and mourning are fully reconciled, they never come up again. Grief comes in and out like the tide. Sometimes heightened periods of sadness occur even years after the death.

Example: My dad loved Frank Sinatra's music—and I have bursts of grief almost every time I hear Frank's voice.

You will always, for the rest of your life, feel some grief over a loved one's death. It will no longer dominate your life, but it will always be there, in the background, reminding you of the love you had for the person who died. And you needn't think of that as a bad thing.

If you follow the advice in this article but are still struggling with grief, consider seeing a compassionate grief counselor. To find one, consult the Association for Death Education and Counseling (ADEC.org).

Index